fP

UNHINGED

THE TROUBLE WITH PSYCHIATRY—
A DOCTOR'S REVELATIONS ABOUT
A PROFESSION IN CRISIS

DANIEL CARLAT

Free Press

New York London Toronto Sydney

fP
FREE PRESS
A Division of Simon & Schuster, Inc.
1230 Avenue of the Americas
New York, NY 10020

The names and details of the patients and other individuals in this book have been changed, and some patients are composites.

First Free Press hardcover edition May 2010

FREE PRESS and colophon are trademarks of Simon & Schuster, Inc.

Manufactured in the United States of America

1 3 5 7 9 10 8 6 4 2

Library of Congress Cataloging-in-Publication Data
Carlat, Daniel J.
Unhinged—the trouble with psychiatry : a doctor's revelations about a profession in crisis / Daniel Carlat. — 1st Free Press hardcover ed.
p. cm.
Includes bibliographical references and index.
1. Psychiatry—Evaluation. 2. Psychotropic drugs. 3. Psychotherapists.
I. Title.
[DNLM: 1. Mental Disorders—therapy. 2. Psychiatry—trends.
3. Psychotherapy—methods. WM 400 C278u 2010]
RC437.5.C3197 2010
616.89—dc22 2009046185

ISBN 978-1-4165-9079-8
ISBN 978-1-4165-9635-6 (ebook)

For my mother, Anita—
May you dance to the end of time.

CONTENTS

UNHINGED

Chapter 1

The Trouble with Psychiatry

For the last fifteen years, I've practiced psychiatry in a small town north of Boston. It is a solo private practice. I see mostly middle-class patients who come to me with depression, anxiety, substance abuse, and occasionally more severe problems, such as bipolar disorder or schizophrenia.

Like most other psychiatrists of my generation, I have specialized in prescribing medications and have referred patients in need of talk treatment to a psychotherapist. During my training at Massachusetts General Hospital, I was taught that we are on the threshold of understanding the biochemistry of mental illness. After I graduated from residency, I worked hard to keep up with the explosion of neuroscience knowledge, and I absorbed the intricacies of how to use the new psychopharmaceuticals as they poured forth from the drug companies at a dizzying clip. By harnessing these powerful medications, I thought I was providing my patients the best psychiatric treatment possible.

But a couple of years ago, I saw a patient who made me question both my profession and my career.

Carol, in her midthirties, had short brown hair and strikingly green eyes that were filled with despair. Once we were seated in my office, I asked her, "How can I be of help?"

"My father was killed in a car accident," she said, choking back tears.

"How awful—when did this happen?"

"Last month."

Carol told me that she had been in the car with her father, who was driving. They came over a rise in the road, and another car was just pulling out of a driveway in front of them. Her father tried to swerve, but it was too late. They collided with the other car, and her father, who was not wearing a seat belt, was killed instantly. Miraculously, Carol was not seriously injured.

Since then, she said, she had recurrent dreams about the accident, and couldn't prevent herself from replaying the scene during the day. The events would unreel themselves like a movie in front of her, and often she would start sobbing uncontrollably. I recognized these experiences—nightmares and flashbacks—as typical symptoms of post-traumatic stress disorder, or PTSD. I asked her a series of questions about other symptoms, such as poor concentration, insomnia, being easily startled, and the need to avoid situations reminding her of the crash, all of which are commonly associated with PTSD.

She said she was experiencing all of them. Her life was constricting inward. She drove rarely, avoiding especially the road where the accident had occurred.

"Are you avoiding anything else?" I asked.

"I won't watch TV. I can't read the newspaper. I never realized how many stories there are about car accidents in the news."

I asked her about symptoms of depression. She reported insomnia and poor motivation, but no suicidal ideation.

"The worst thing," she said, "is how guilty I feel."

"Why guilty?" I asked.

"It was my fault that we crashed. I got him upset."

Her eyes began to well up. "I was telling him that he shouldn't be drinking."

"He was drinking and driving?"

She nodded. "I told him I could smell it on his breath and that he shouldn't be driving. He got mad, started yelling at me. And then he floored the gas pedal, said something like 'Am I driving good enough now?' That's when it happened."

I could see that this was more than a simple case of PTSD. She would have complicated feelings about her father to wrestle with—grief, regret, and eventually a good deal of anger.

As the end of the hour approached, I told her a bit about PTSD, about the prognosis for recovery, and about the usual treatments.

"So what do you think I should do?" she asked me.

"I'd like to give you some medication to help you through this," I said. I wrote out prescriptions for the antidepressant Zoloft and for the tranquilizer Klonopin. Then I reached into my file cabinet, and handed her a business card. "And this is a good therapist who I often work with. I recommend that you give her a call and set up an appointment. The medication works better when you are also seeing a counselor."

She looked confused. "Aren't *you* my therapist?"

I shook my head. "Unfortunately, I don't have time in my practice to do therapy. I usually refer patients to psychotherapists whom I trust."

"So . . . am I going to see you again?"

"Yes, we'll schedule another appointment in about a month, to see how the medications are working. But in the meantime, I hope you'll have had a couple of sessions with this other doctor."

Carol still didn't look at all happy with this.

"But aren't there any psychiatrists that do therapy?"

"There are a few," I said, "but not many. They're hard to find these days."

After Carol left my office, I finished writing her intake note. I closed her chart, put my pen down, and looked out my office window at the white-steepled Unitarian church across the street. There was nothing unusual about my encounter with Carol. I did what most psychiatrists do when they encounter a new patient. I sat comfortably in my red leather chair, wearing my suit and tie, and I asked her a series of diagnostic questions. Her answers fit neatly into a recipe book of psychiatric diagnoses called the DSM-IV (Diagnostic and Statistical Manual of Mental Disorders, fourth edition), and I pieced together a diagnosis that made sense to me. I then reached over to my desk, wrote out a prescription, and handed it to her.

Pondering this typical appointment, what struck me most was what I did *not* do. I am an MD, having gone through four years of medical school, one year of grueling medical internship in a general hospital, and three years of psychiatric residency at Massachusetts General Hospital. But, like most psychiatrists, I did little to take advantage of those years of training. I did not do a physical exam, nor did I take Carol's pulse or blood pressure. Indeed, the only times I stirred from my chair were to meet her in the waiting room at the beginning and to show her into my secretary's office to make a follow-up appointment at the end.

Just as striking to me as the lack of typical doctorly activities in psychiatry is the dearth of psychotherapy. Most people are under the misconception that an appointment with a psychiatrist will involve counseling, probing questions, and digging into the psychological meanings of one's distress. But the psychiatrist as psychotherapist is an endangered species. In fact, according to the latest data from a group of researchers at Columbia University, only one out of every ten psychiatrists offers therapy to all their patients.[1] Doing psychotherapy doesn't pay well enough. I can see three or four patients per hour if I focus on medications (such psychiatrists are called "psychopharmacologists"), but only one patient in that time period if I do therapy. The income differential is a powerful incentive to drop therapy from our repertoire of skills, and psychiatrists have generally followed the money.

So, like most of my patients, Carol saw me for medications, and saw a social worker colleague for therapy. Her symptoms gradually improved, but whether this was due to the medications or the therapy, or simply the passage of time, I cannot say.

Carol's treatment was not particularly dramatic, but her story illustrates both the triumphs and the failures of modern psychiatry. Over the last thirty years, we have constructed a reliable system for diagnosing mental disorders, and we have created medications that work well to treat a range of psychological symptoms. But these very successes have had unpredictable consequences. As psychiatrists have become enthralled with diagnosis and medication, we have given up the essence of our profession—understanding the mind. We have become obsessed with psychopharmacology and its endless process of tinkering with medications, adjusting dosages, and piling on more medications to treat the side effects of the drugs we started with. We have convinced ourselves that we have developed cures for mental illnesses like Carol's, when in fact we know so little about the underlying neurobiology of their causes that our treatments are often a series of trials and errors.

Theories of the neurobiology of PTSD, depression, and the range of other mental illnesses have come and gone over the years, but we are still far away from a true understanding of the biological causes of these diseases. Clearly, thoughts and emotions arise from the activity of neurons, and it makes sense that when emotions are distorted severely, the neurons must in some way be "broken." Theories about depression over the years have included different versions of the "chemical imbalance" idea. The 2009 version of the American Psychiatric Association's *Textbook of Psychopharmacology* reviews these candidate chemicals in depth.[2] Researchers have found evidence of abnormalities in serotonin, norepinephrine, dopamine, cortisol, thyroid, growth hormone, glutamate, and brain-derived neurotrophic factor—yet no specific defect has been identified. Straying outside the world of chemistry, other researchers have tried to find the causes of depression through neuroimaging scans. But this research has been just as inconclusive. Some of the major findings include decreased activity in the left frontal lobe, a shrunken hippocampus, an oversized amygdala, disrupted circuits around the basal ganglia, and miscellaneous abnormalities in the thalamus and the pituitary gland.

The APA textbook authors, utterly unable to tie together these disparate findings, concluded that the "central question of what variables drive the pathophysiology of mood disorders remains unanswered." You can say that again. The problem is not in the enthusiasm or intelligence of the researchers—but rather in the inherent complexity of the brain itself. A typical brain contains one hundred billion neurons, each of which makes electrical connections, or synapses, with up to ten thousand other neurons. That means a *quadrillion* synapses are active at any given time—the number of people on 150,000 Earths. It is therefore no surprise that we know almost nothing definitive about the pathophysiology of mental illness—the surprise is that we know anything at all.

While the scientific literature contains thousands of papers proposing neurobiological theories to explain PTSD, depression, bipolar disorder, schizophrenia, and other psychiatric disorders, these theories remain unproven, and they are rarely based on an in-depth understanding of how the brain works. Instead, researchers generate these theories by working backward from having discovered that a certain drug seems to be effective in treating a disease's symptoms. Thus, the fact that many antidepressants increase levels of serotonin has led to a serotonin-deficiency theory of depression, even though direct evidence of such a deficiency is lacking. By this same logic one could argue that the cause of all pain conditions is a deficiency of opiates, since narcotic pain medications activate opiate receptors in the brain. In fact, pain is caused by a multitude of mechanisms, depending on which organ is involved. Chest pain from a heart attack is not caused by an opiate deficiency, for example, but by a lack of blood flow to certain cardiac tissues, which damages heart cells. This is a true physiological explanation of a disease, one that has guided the development of cardiac medications that act by increasing blood flow to the heart muscle. By contrast, the shocking truth is that psychiatry has yet to develop a convincing explanation for the pathophysiology of any illness at all.

Psychiatry's scientific failures were encapsulated recently by none other than the country's chief psychiatrist, Dr. Thomas Insel, the head of the National Institute of Mental Health. In an editorial recently published in one of the top psychiatric journals, Insel summed up the primitive state of psychiatric knowledge this way: "Despite high expectations, neither genomics nor imaging has yet impacted the diagnosis or treatment of the 45 million Americans with serious or moderate mental illness each year." He added: "While we have seen profound progress in research . . . the gap between the surge in basic biological knowledge and the state of mental health care in this country has not narrowed and may be getting wider."[3]

The science of psychiatry is riveting, and I have confidence that someday we will understand the neurobiology of emotions, and come up with effective treatments based on that knowledge. But we are much further away from this understanding than most of my patients think. Patients often view psychiatrists as wizards of neurotransmitters, who can choose just the right medication for whatever chemical imbalance is at play. This exaggerated conception of our capabilities has been encouraged by drug companies, by psychiatrists ourselves, and by our patients' understandable hopes for cures.

In medical school, there's an old joke that goes like this: Internists know everything and do nothing, surgeons know nothing and do everything, pathologists know everything and do everything (but a day too late), and psychiatrists know nothing and do nothing. The punch line is particularly insulting to psychiatrists, and it is not really accurate. We know *some*thing and we do *some*thing, but we know and we do far less than we might care to admit.

Before his untimely death by suicide at forty-six, David Foster Wallace was considered by many to be the most brilliant novelist of his generation. His 1996 masterpiece, *Infinite Jest*, was a satirical futuristic novel whose plot concerns a movie called *Infinite Jest* that people find so entertaining and alluring that they sit for days watching it, becoming paralyzed and lifeless.[4] A 1,097-page reflection on the nature of modern entertainment, it became a sensation, winning Wallace a cultlike following, and was eventually included by *Time* magazine in its list of "100 Best English-language Novels from 1923 to 2005."

But Wallace could hardly enjoy his achievements and his fame, because he suffered from chronic depression and anxiety. The history of his treatment has been chronicled recently in both *The New Yorker*[5] and *Rolling Stone*[6] magazines, and these accounts give a disquieting glimpse into the limits of modern psychiatry.

Wallace first suffered depression as an undergraduate at Amherst College, and in a story he wrote for Amherst's literary magazine, he provided a vivid picture of his suffering:

> You are the sickness yourself. . . . You realize all this . . . when you look at the black hole and it's wearing your face. That's when the Bad Thing just absolutely eats you up, or rather when you just eat yourself up. When you kill yourself. All this business about people committing suicide when they're "severely depressed": we say, "Holy cow, we must do something to stop them from killing themselves!" That's wrong. Because all these people have, you see, by this time already killed themselves, where it really counts. . . . When they "commit suicide," they're just being orderly.

Wallace sought treatment and was prescribed a tricyclic, an older type of medication that was the first effective antidepressant to be developed, but he stopped after two months, later telling a journalist that the medication "made me feel like I was stoned and in hell." Presumably, he was referring to the sedation and other side effects common with tricyclics.

During graduate school at Harvard, Wallace dealt with depression by escaping into alcohol and drug use. Eventually, frightened by escalating thoughts of suicide, he again consulted a psychiatrist, resulting in an eight-day psychiatric admission to McLean Hospital (a hospital where I did a bit of training, since it is affiliated with Mass General). At McLean, according to his mother, "we had a brief, maybe three-minute audience with the psychopharmacologist," and Wallace was prescribed Nardil, another old but quite potent antidepressant, one that requires a special diet devoid of certain cheeses and cured meats.

Nardil worked fairly well for Wallace. Though he still suffered periods of depression and anxiety, he was able to live his life, continue his writing, and get married. In June 2007, however, he ate a meal at an Indian restaurant that caused him days of stomach cramping, and doctors thought the symptoms might have been caused by an interaction of the food with the drug. Tired of having to worry about the many side effects of Nardil, and having been on the drug for almost two decades, he decided, in cooperation with his psychiatrists, to try to stop it.

Coming off Nardil certainly seemed a reasonable decision. By then, drug companies had produced dozens of newer drugs to treat his symptoms, with far fewer side effects than MAOIs (monoamine oxidase inhibitors, the class of drug to which Nardil belonged). Wallace was tapered off the Nardil and tried on a succession of newer antidepressants. While we don't know the details, from my own experience treating patients with chronic depression I can imagine how his treatment proceeded. His psychiatrist likely rotated through a series of drugs, going from one mechanism of action to another, using combinations of drugs, possibly adding lithium, thyroid, or an antipsychotic to "augment" the effects of other drugs. Nothing worked. Whatever was tried, Wallace remained depressed, and after a year of different drug trials, he was put back on Nardil. But as sometimes happens when a once-effective drug is reintroduced, Nardil had lost its potency. Desperate, Wallace eventually agreed to electric shock therapy, which famously cured the depression of Kitty Dukakis, the wife of the 1988 Democratic presidential nominee, Michael Dukakis.[7] But it didn't work for Wallace. One night, at the end of August 2008, his wife left him at home alone for a few hours, and when she returned, he had hung himself.

In any field of medicine, patients become desperately ill and die before their time, despite the best efforts of doctors. This is as true in cardiology and oncology as it is in psychiatry. Wallace's story does not imply that psychiatry is ineffective, but his failure to respond to any drug other than Nardil—which was introduced in the 1950s—illustrates a sad truth about our medications. Whether we are talking about depression, schizophrenia, or bipolar disorder, the new drugs introduced over the past fifty years are no more effective than the original prototypes—such as Haldol for schizophrenia, lithium for bipolar disorder, and Nardil for depression. We are keen to prescribe the newest drugs, and patients assume that much progress has been made in psychopharmacology over the past several decades, but as I'll explore more fully later, this progress has been overblown.

This frustrating reality has recently been demonstrated by several large studies that were not funded by drug companies, and were therefore not biased in their research designs to favor particular drugs. These studies, conducted by the National Institute of Mental Health and known by various acronyms such as the CATIE trial, the STAR-D trial, and the STEP-BD trial, have demonstrated that the newer drugs for schizophrenia, depression, and bipolar disorder are generally no more effective than the older drugs they have largely replaced.[8] Furthermore, even our newer drugs' supposed advantage—fewer side effects—is being called into question. For example, the original antipsychotics such as Haldol and Thorazine sometimes caused permanent neurological side effects, which are largely avoided by the newer "atypical" antipsychotics, such as Zyprexa, Risperdal, and Seroquel. But research has shown that these newer agents cause problems of their own, such as obesity, diabetes, and cardiovascular disease.[9]

Because of this, the progress of psychiatry over the second half of the twentieth century has been less dramatic than commonly portrayed. We have witnessed a steady accumulation of new drugs, but "new" has not always meant "better." This explosion of products led to the emergence of an entirely new subdiscipline of psychiatry called "psychopharmacology," the specialization in prescribing medications, and psychopharmacologists rarely do therapy. This new discipline ushered in, in therapy's place, the "fifteen-minute med check." Such short visits were unheard of thirty years ago, but have now become the defining appointment of modern practitioners. Meanwhile, the psychotherapy skills of many psychiatrists have largely withered away, if they were ever taught to them in the first place.

There was a time when I thought this shift in the profession was a natural evolution. Why put patients through months and years of weekly therapy if simply taking pills worked as well if not better? As it turns out, we were wrong in two ways. We both exaggerated the effectiveness of the new drugs and gave psychotherapy a premature burial.

Linda, a woman in her forties, came to see me a couple of years ago because she had been feeling increasingly discouraged with her life. Her husband was disabled with a cardiac condition and she needed to look after him constantly. Their marriage was filled with conflict, and each day felt like a long argument. Linda wanted to leave her husband, but felt trapped, too guilty to leave him in his time of greatest need.

Her desperation leeched into the rest of her life. Most mornings she woke up both exhausted and anxious. She felt hopeless and regretful of her life decisions. Of greatest concern to me, she had begun to wish she could "just disappear," although she assured me that she had neither the desire nor the "courage" to actually harm herself.

At the end of my customary fifty-minute diagnostic evaluation, I told Linda that I thought she was suffering from major depression, and recommended a medication that might help. I said that I had good experience with Lexapro, an antidepressant in the category of SSRIs (selective serotonin reuptake inhibitors). She wondered why I chose this particular drug, and I explained that Lexapro worked by increasing the amount of serotonin in the brain, and it seemed to have fewer side effects than other antidepressants. She took the prescription, and I booked a follow-up appointment with her for a month later, which was the soonest I had an opening. I told her that I did not have room in my schedule to see her for psychotherapy sessions, but I gave her the names of two good counselors I knew.

After she left, as I did with my patient Carol, I reflected on several things that I did not tell Linda.

I didn't tell her that, despite my training at Harvard's Massachusetts General Hospital, I have no idea how Lexapro works to relieve depression, nor does any other psychiatrist. Like the Zoloft I had given Carol, while Lexapro increases levels of serotonin in the nerve synapses, there is no direct evidence that depression is a disorder of reduced serotonin. The term "chemical imbalance" is commonly used by laypeople as a shorthand explanation for mental illness. It is a convenient myth because it destigmatizes their condition—if the problem is a chemical imbalance, it is not their fault. Psychiatrists go along with this shorthand, because it gives us something to say when patients ask us questions about pathophysiology. After all, no doctor wants to admit ignorance about the very problems he or she is trained to manage.

I did not tell Linda that psychotherapy might work just as well as medication for her, and that I had decided on medication in part because I received little training in therapy during my three years of psychiatric residency. Like many psychiatrists, I *don't* do psychotherapy because I *can't* do psychotherapy.

I did not ask Linda to have her blood drawn, nor did I send her for a brain scan. Diagnosis in psychiatry proceeds exactly as it did a century ago—by asking a series of questions and analyzing the responses. Patients often ask us for a "diagnostic test." They hear media reports about PET scans, EEGs, and computerized tests of attention. Both psychiatrists and their patients are quick to embrace these talismans of hard science, but, unfortunately, psychiatric diagnosis continues to lag far behind the rest of medicine. Because of this, the DSM-IV, our diagnostic manual, has taken on the dimensions of a holy book in the field. Every ten years or so, a new edition is published, and the landscape of psychiatry changes. But, as I'll show later, the new diagnoses are based on votes of committees of psychiatrists, rather than neurobiological testing. Because diagnosis in psychiatry is more art than science, the field is vulnerable to "disease mongering," the expansion of disease definitions in order to pump up the market for medication treatment.

Finally, I did not tell Linda that I was often visited by a pharmaceutical representative from Forest Pharmaceuticals, the maker of Lexapro, who would bring me my favorite drink from Starbucks and sandwiches for my receptionist. The rep had told me that Lexapro was the best tolerated of all SSRIs, and while I knew that there is no convincing evidence that this is true, her visit accomplished its objective, which was to plant Lexapro uppermost in my mind. And I, in turn, prescribed it to Linda.

I continued to see Linda for another year or so. She had many side effects on medications, and so I rotated her through different treatments, relying on trial and error because there is little else to guide our prescribing decisions. She felt a little better than when I had first seen her. As often happens in my field, Linda eventually disappeared from my practice. She simply stopped making appointments. I had no reason to believe that she disliked me or was unhappy with my care. But as is common in psychiatry, we had developed no strong therapeutic connection over the course of fifteen-minute visits every other month. Wherever she is, I hope she is doing well.

Like my patient Carol, there was nothing extraordinary about Linda. On the contrary, she is representative of the broad number of patients my colleagues and I see regularly—and she illustrates what is wrong with the profession of psychiatry in the twenty-first century.

Psychiatrists, who as recently as thirty years ago saw patients for hour-long sessions, often several times per week, have become so tightly scheduled with fifteen-minute so-called sessions that we have little or no time for therapy anymore. Our diagnostic process is shallow and is based on an elaborate checklist of symptoms, leading us sometimes to overdiagnose patients with disorders of questionable validity, or, conversely, to miss the underlying problems in our rush to come up with a discrete diagnostic label that will be reimbursed by the insurance company. We tend to treat all psychological problems the same way—with a pill and a few words of encouragement. Because of this rote approach to treatment, patients are often misdiagnosed and medications are overprescribed. In the end, we misserve our patients, failing to offer them psychotherapies that are sometimes more effective than drugs.

We have been seduced by the constant encouragement from drug companies to prescribe more medications and an insurance reimbursement system that discourages therapy. On top of these inducements, an outmoded training regimen in medical school provides years of unneeded courses in surgery and internal medicine while providing little training in the specific skills needed by psychiatrists.

Pulled by both drug companies and consumer demand to provide immediate drug fixes to life's difficulties, the field of psychiatry has become unhinged, pried away from its original mission—to discover the causes of mental illness and to treat those causes, not merely the symptoms. At a time when direct-to-consumer drug advertising has tripled in the last ten years, from $1.3 billion in 1999 to $4.8 billion in 2008, blockbuster drugs that promise to treat symptoms such as shyness (Paxil), fatigue (Provigil), stage fright (the generic drug propranolol), and sexual problems (Viagra) have become rooted in the public consciousness.[10] Sometimes the drugs work well, and sometimes they do little but cause side effects. Nonetheless, the going narrative is that psychiatry has a biochemical solution for every variant of distress. This story yields profits for drug companies, prestige for psychiatrists, and reassurance for patients. But the narrative is full of holes.

In *Unhinged*, I will take you on a guided tour of the landscape of modern psychiatry. I will show you what we actually know about the mind—versus what we only pretend to know. I will argue that we psychiatrists spend our days splitting our patients into two: one is a repository of neurotransmitters, and the other is a person with relationships, a job, and aspirations. We treat the neurotransmitters, and we refer the person to somebody else.

The surprise is that our treatments are remarkably helpful to patients, even though we hobble ourselves in this way. Imagine how effective we could be if we embraced all the tools at our disposal. This is my ultimate goal in *Unhinged*—to envision a different kind of psychiatrist, and to provide a road map for achieving this vision.

Chapter 2

On Becoming a Psychiatrist

My own training began just as psychiatry was in the midst of its transformation from psychotherapy to psychopharmacology. In 1985, three years before the introduction of Prozac, I started medical school at the University of California at San Francisco, with the goal of eventually becoming a psychiatrist. People are often curious, even suspicious, about why psychiatrists choose their profession. I was always interested in the human psyche, and knew that I would become either a psychiatrist or a psychologist. The difference between the two is that psychiatrists go to medical school and can prescribe drugs, whereas psychologists go to graduate school and learn about therapy and research methods, and, with the recent exception of two states,[1] cannot prescribe medication. My father is a psychiatrist, and he advised me to go to medical school—and not only because he wanted to see his son following in his footsteps. He has collaborated with psychologists for years and found that some were frustrated by not being able to prescribe medications. He wanted me to avoid that same potential frustration.

But there was a darker side to my career decision. My mother suffered severe mental illness, with debilitating depressions and paranoid thoughts. One autumn day during my junior year in college, she committed suicide.

Unlike David Foster Wallace, my mother had not been in treatment for most of her life. In fact, the extent of her troubles was not even clear to me until after her death. My parents had divorced when I was five, and I lived with my mother until high school. She was generally a high-spirited, fun-loving person, but I recall days when she had little energy and spent many hours sleeping. If I had been her psychiatrist, I might have diagnosed her with major depression or bipolar disorder. Whatever her diagnostic label, she managed to keep her full-time job as a nurse, maintained a household, and took good care of me, her only child.

However, there were early hints of problems to come. For example, I recall a few times when she was convinced that our apartment had been bugged with listening devices, but as a ten-year-old, it never occurred to me to think that she was "crazy." During the late sixties many people believed that the FBI kept files on just about any American who might be identified as a leftist activist, and my mother certainly qualified, having been actively involved in the National Organization for Women. There was a cultural context for her paranoia, and I'm not certain that it would necessarily have been considered a "delusion" at the time. She behaved rationally otherwise, never had hallucinations that I knew of, and, at any rate, life seemed to proceed fairly normally despite her idiosyncratic beliefs.

But soon after I started college at U.C. Berkeley, she worsened. Reconstructing events, at some point she moved back to the small town in Pennsylvania where she grew up, and told her family that agents from the Montgomery Ward department store had been on her plane in order to monitor her. She was admitted to a psychiatric hospital with depression and paranoid delusions, and killed herself some time after her discharge.

As a twenty-year-old, I found her suicide to be absolutely devastating, and it taught me how much pain a suicide inflicts on the surviving family. I make use of this knowledge to help my suicidal patients now, making a point to discuss with them the potential impact on their families. Her suicide also cemented my desire to go into psychiatry, and eventually I was admitted to medical school.

Medical school is a challenging rite of passage for anyone, but for those few who use it as a ticket to psychiatry, it is particularly brutal. My goal was to penetrate the mysteries of the mind, but instead I found myself memorizing intricacies of biochemistry, such as the Krebs Cycle, that I would never apply in my psychiatric practice. Rather than absorbing the theories of psychotherapy, I learned about kidneys, acid/base balances, and cardiac contractility. And like medical students through the ages, I put in my hours in the gross anatomy lab, cutting through leathery skin, peering into dead organs, and tracing the paths of arteries and nerves.

After these classroom courses, I started my clinical rotations, which are mini-apprenticeships in the different medical specialties. Each rotation lasted from one to two months, and they took place at different hospitals affiliated with the University of California at San Francisco. My first rotation was at the San Francisco V.A. Medical Center. Morning rounds began at 6 a.m. (sharp!) in the vascular surgery unit. Most of the patients were severe diabetics whose disease had virtually cut off the blood supply to their legs. Consequently, gangrene set in, requiring amputations and vigilant post-op wound care to prevent further loss of limb. During rounds, a group of medical students and the attending visited each patient, clustering around freshly cut stumps to learn how to determine whether the wounds had the healthy red granularity of healing tissue or the foul-smelling yellowish sheen of oxygen-starved cells.

Fatigued and nauseated, I tried to generate a facsimile of enthusiasm as we drifted from bed to bed. But my mind was elsewhere, wondering if I had made a mistake choosing medical school rather than a program in clinical psychology. My first intensive immersion in psychiatry came in my fourth year, and it yielded two major lessons. First, it confirmed that I had chosen the right field, because for the first time in my medical career I was riveted by the clinical work. But second, it demonstrated for me that the underlying science of psychiatry was in a shockingly primitive state in comparison with the rest of medicine.

I was assigned to one of the inpatient units at Langley Porter Neuropsychiatric Hospital. Most of the patients had schizophrenia, bipolar disorder, or severe depression and had been brought to the hospital by the police because they were dangerous to themselves or to others. I recall one patient, a man with flowing red hair and a messianic beard, who was admitted after the police found him doing cartwheels on the highway during rush hour. He was acting under the delusion that he was Jesus Christ and was therefore invincible. Another patient was convinced that her parents had been replaced by "imposters" who looked and behaved very much like her real parents, but who were dangerous. She was brought to the hospital because she said that these imposters needed to be killed. This strange delusion is not uncommon, and has been given a name: Capgras syndrome.

Upon admission, each patient received a full medical workup, which typically included a CT scan of the brain and a series of blood tests. But the results of the tests were virtually always normal; when there were abnormalities, they reflected medical illnesses unrelated to the psychiatric issue, such as diabetes or cardiac illness. We did physical exams as well, but like the lab tests, the purpose was to rule out a medical illness rather than to diagnose a psychiatric one.[2]

The process of psychiatric diagnosis was strikingly different from what I had been exposed to during my medical and surgical rotations. For example, in medicine a patient might be admitted with severe shortness of breath and we would take a quick history, listen urgently to the heart and lungs, get a measure of oxygen saturation, and review X-rays and blood tests in order to distinguish among cardiac disease, lung disease, and infection. These various physiological measurements were crucial to determining both the diagnosis and the treatment.

In psychiatry, on the other hand, the physical exams and blood tests seemed rote exercises done for medico-legal reasons. Nobody wanted to be sued for missing a brain tumor, even though the possibility of a brain tumor causing psychiatric symptoms without any obvious physical symptoms is remote. The results rarely influenced diagnosis or treatment. Psychosis, violent thoughts, depression—all these symptoms were ascertained strictly by conversing with a patient. And the causes of the symptoms, at least on a neurobiological level, were simply unknown.

I began to learn in more detail about the limitations of psychiatric science with my very first patient, Dave, a twenty-one-year-old college junior who had been admitted to the hospital after a Tylenol overdose. Ironically, Tylenol, a nostrum for mild aches and pains that is available to anyone over the counter, is one of the most lethal of medications when taken in overdose. In high concentrations, one of its metabolites rapidly destroys the tissues of the liver, leading potentially to coma and death. Dave was lucky in that he was brought to the hospital soon after he overdosed, and was given an antidote that prevented significant liver damage. After he recovered in the intensive care unit, he was transferred to the locked part of the psychiatric ward, where he was started on an antidepressant and was put on a suicide watch.

I found Dave in his room. He had brown hair and brown eyes, and was dressed in a T-shirt, khaki shorts, and flip-flops. What struck me immediately was how normal he looked. Though he was a few years younger than I, I could have easily imagined him as a classmate or a friend, someone to play tennis with or to hang out with in a café.

He smiled as I greeted him, but he had a pained look in his eyes that communicated embarrassment as much as depression. "I don't really belong in places like this," his expression seemed to say. This was hardly my image of a suicidal patient. I had been expecting someone decidedly less preppy, maybe with stringy black hair and pale skin and dirty jeans.

He followed me down the carpeted hallway into the interview room, where we pulled up two chairs. He sat with his elbows on his knees and his head hanging down. As we talked, he sometimes looked up at me with his sad eyes and forced a smile.

Speaking quietly, he told me that his depression had been triggered by girlfriend problems—personality incompatibilities, arguments about movie choices, and disagreements about the future. They broke up, then got back together, but still couldn't seem to hit a stride in their relationship. It was during this time that Dave overdosed.

As I listened to his story, I had that same uncanny sense of normality. I could identify with his girlfriend problems and the seemingly trivial arguments that cause a relationship to peter out. I'd been through such relationships in college and medical school. I'd experienced the lingering pain of on again/off again relationships. But I had never jumped the chasm from that pain to feeling suicidal.

There was a pause, and I asked him why he had felt so bad about the situation. He shook his head, his gaze still fixed to the floor. "I disappointed so many people. My family, my girlfriend. It was all my fault."

"Why was it your fault?"

"Because I lied about things."

"What sorts of things?"

"About my feelings. I thought I loved her, but I don't think I can love anyone. I don't deserve anything. I don't deserve to live."

"Dave," I said, "I'm trying to understand exactly what you did that was so awful that you felt you deserved to be dead. I just don't get it."

But Dave continued to simply declare that he was a "bad" person.

When I spoke with his parents and girlfriend, they described Dave as having always been moody, but also kind and compassionate. Far from being "bad," they told me, Dave was deeply religious.

I wondered whether Dave's unexplained "guilt" had to do with his religion.

"Do you feel that God is punishing you for something?" I asked.

"Of course he is," he responded with fervor. "I've disappointed him profoundly. Look at me . . . look at where I am." He waved toward the nurse's station and the hallway beyond, where patients were lining up to receive their medications. "This is where I've ended up. I don't have a job. I don't have anyplace to live. I've failed him miserably."

"But don't you think God forgives you? Don't you think he loves you unconditionally?"

He shook his head. "I don't know."

We ordered the usual series of lab tests, but they were all normal. The only abnormality on his physical exam, ironically, was one that we had caused by our treatment. His antidepressant, nortriptyline, caused a blood pressure problem called "orthostatic hypotension," which prevents the normal transient increase in blood pressure when patients stand up quickly. So Dave became dizzy if he stood up quickly, and once nearly fainted.

Nortriptyline was supposed to help Dave by increasing levels of both serotonin and norepinephrine, but whether Dave suffered from a chemical imbalance, as this notion was based on, or some other, yet-to-be-determined defect, he was not improving despite high doses of the drug. We were particularly discouraged when one day he revealed to us that he had been hoarding some of his pills with a plan to attempt suicide again. Thereafter, the nursing staff did mouth checks to make sure he swallowed his pills, but still he did not improve. Because his guilt was so extreme as to border on the delusional, we gave him the antipsychotic Haldol, but this only served to make him sleepy. The attending began broaching the topic of electroconvulsive therapy, often more effective than medications in psychotic depression, but Dave was reluctant because of the possible side effect of memory loss.

We tried to provide psychotherapy as well, but Dave's depression was so severe that his neurons seemed to be firing through molasses. He responded to questions slowly, and it was hard to sort out the logic of his depression, if indeed there was a logic. I saw my role as a hand-holder, as someone to gently coach him through his hospitalization. At times, when we felt he was safe, we gave him passes to go on outings with his family. Once, he made the mistake of seeing his ex-girlfriend on a pass and this set him back.

My rotation on the psych unit lasted for six weeks, and on my last day, when I said my good-byes, Dave was still on round-the-clock suicide checks. In team meetings, we discussed other medication combinations to try. We thought about having a hospital chaplain visit with him to help him make more positive use of his faith. Mostly, we were very frustrated with our inability to do much more than provide a safe place for him. For some patients, the best we can do is to keep them alive and hope that something changes within them to ease their suffering.

Somewhere, presumably, encased within his skull, neural circuits were misfiring, keeping him paralyzed in a quasi-life. But nobody knew what those circuits might be, let alone had any idea how they might be repaired. Two years later, when I arrived in Boston to begin my psychiatry residency at Massachusetts General Hospital, I joined a group of psychiatrists who believed this knowledge was just around the corner.

* * *

Massachusetts General Hospital is an impressive sight when glimpsed from Cambridge Street, looking north to the White Building. It is all hospital—humming with medical energy, ambulances screeching up to the ER, patients looking for their appointments, and battalions of health care personnel making their way to their departments.

I began my residency on a sweltering, sticky day in mid-July. My first rotation was on the inpatient unit, Bullfinch 3, and I took my place in the hierarchy of a clinical team, consisting of myself, the attending physician, a nurse, a social worker, and a psychology intern. I interviewed patients in the mornings and would later meet with the team to come up with a treatment plan.

The unit held twenty patients, and the four residents split up the patient load, meaning that I was typically responsible for treating five patients. When they were admitted, I would do the initial workup, including a diagnostic interview and physical exam. The attendings saw all patients as well, but relied on the residents to gather most of the information. The most common diagnosis was depression, with a smattering of patients with disorders such as Alzheimer's dementia, eating disorders, and schizophrenia. All patients received medications, and some received ECT, or shock therapy, for depression. Often, patients were on combinations of four or five psychiatric medications, with more medications to treat drug side effects like constipation or tremor.

The year was 1992, and clearly psychopharmacology was in ascendance. America was becoming "Prozac nation," and many of the key clinical trials for the newer antidepressants had been conducted by MGH psychiatrists. These faculty members commanded millions of dollars in grants from both drug companies and government sources and walked around the hospital with a confident swagger. Nonetheless, I soon detected tensions between attendings who were therapy advocates versus those who relied more on drugs to treat patients.

This issue surfaced in the case of one patient, thirty-year-old William, who had shown up in the emergency room paranoid and depressed. A junior executive at a financial firm, William said that he had a long-term relationship with his girlfriend, but when she went away on a long trip with her family, he met another woman. "I fell in love," he told me. "I fell hard." Unfortunately, she decided to break up with him, and the morning after the breakup, William found himself at his desk at work unable to concentrate, crying, shaking, and having an uncanny feeling that everybody around him was an enemy. A coworker drove him to the emergency room, and he was admitted with the initial diagnosis of "brief psychotic disorder," a somewhat noncommittal label to describe what William colloquially termed a "nervous breakdown."[3]

Reading the nurse's notes before going into his room to introduce myself, I was struck that this was not only his first psychiatric admission, but also his first psychiatric treatment of any kind. I wondered how someone could go through life apparently healthy for thirty years, and then fall apart so completely.

I found William sitting at the small desk in his room. He was dressed in a white button-down shirt, monogrammed on the pocket with his initials, and brown corduroys. His face was very tan and surreally handsome, as if somebody had been able to shop for the best elements of a face and had put them all together. A strong chin, blue eyes, casually tossed brown hair, perfect teeth. He was reading a book about financial securities.

I introduced myself, and rather than shaking my hand, his eyes narrowed, and he said: "Are you a real doctor or just a resident?"

Thrown off guard, I said, "I'm a resident, but I work under the attending, and I *am* a real—"

"Why can't I speak to the attending?" He interrupted me. "I know how the system works in these places. I'm a 'training case,' right? How many patients have you seen?"

I was rattled, but eventually I got William to agree to talk to me as long as I promised that he would also have a chance to meet with the attending. He told me that he had been depressed for a long time, because he could never find the "right" person to be with. "I have high standards," he said. "And this new woman appeared to meet all of them. Now I have nothing." I asked him about his girlfriend. "She doesn't know about this, but I assume it's over with her. That doesn't bother me. She had problems."

During the team meeting, we decided to start him on a combination of medications to target each of his symptoms: an antidepressant for his sadness, an antipsychotic for the paranoia, and a sleeping pill for his insomnia. But the following day, a Saturday, the on-call attending, Dr. F., hearing the story from me, said, "This guy sounds like he has narcissistic personality disorder. I doubt the meds are going to do much. Why don't you bring him in and let me talk to him."

Narcissistic personality disorder is named after Narcissus, the youth from Greek and Roman mythology who falls in love with his own reflection in a pool. While the term narcissistic is commonly used to describe people who believe they are better than everybody else, in psychiatric terms, it refers to patients who unconsciously believe they are defective and deeply flawed. In order to mask their self-hatred, they develop a veneer of false confidence and superiority over others. Often, this takes the form of being highly critical and setting up impossibly high standards for people in their lives. But this only serves to alienate others, leading to rejection, loneliness, and sometimes suicidal depression.[4]

Dr. F. was in his seventies and never hesitated to speak his mind. Unlike many of the psychiatrists in the department, Dr. F. had few academic aspirations, and had been hired more for his extraordinary clinical skills rather than for his potential as a researcher. He worked at Bullfinch in the mornings and maintained a busy private practice in the afternoons. His philosophy of treatment was "do or say whatever you need to do to get the patient better." Sometimes that meant medication, sometimes it meant therapy. He believed that since hospital stays were so short, you had to very quickly get to the bottom of their psychological issues and confront them, hopefully giving patients something important to ponder as they continued their outpatient treatment after discharge.

I asked William to come into the conference room, and I introduced him to Dr. F., who shook his hand, smiled, and said, "Dr. Carlat has told me a little about you. It sounds like you've had a hard time finding the right woman. What are the obstacles?"

"No one has the right qualities, like morality and courage."

"Your standards are high," observed Dr. F.

"Extremely."

"And now you feel lonely. You are someone who needs somebody to love." Dr. F. was leaning forward, gazing directly into William's eyes.

"Of course I do," he responded, looking impatient.

"It's a paradox," said Dr. F. "You hold yourself out as yearning to have people in your life. But almost no one has met your standards."

"I guess not."

"You apply those standards to yourself also, don't you?"

"Yes."

"So I'd worry that you would hold yourself in contempt."

"I feel like a failure. I've masked it by being a high achiever."

After a few seconds of silence, Dr. F. leaned back in his chair.

"William," he said, "I'd like you to spend some of your time here on the unit looking at what the real problem is. Is it truly that you can't find the right person? Or is it that you've set your standards so high that you have contempt for everyone, including yourself?"

William appeared to be pondering these words, but then said,

"With all due respect, doctor, I think you're off base here. Are you the head of the department?"

"No, I'm one of the attendings on the unit."

"Well," he said, "I'd like to get a second opinion from someone a little more senior. So far, I've talked to a resident"—he pointed at me—"and now a staff psychiatrist. I had expected a little more. Isn't this a Harvard hospital?"

Now William was treating Dr. F. just as he had treated me. At least he was an equal opportunity narcissist! I was curious to see how my teacher would handle William's confrontation.

Dr. F. leaned forward. "This is what you do out there, isn't it?"

"What are you talking about?"

"When somebody threatens your self-esteem, as I fear I just did when I tried to diagnose your issues, you react by demeaning them, and I'd imagine this leads you to be a lonely person."

"Look—I was just pointing out that I deserve a second opinion."

"That's right, and in the process you managed to insult both Dr. Carlat and me. That's okay. We can take it. Our job is to put up a mirror and show you what you do in your life, and how your patterns led you to be in the hospital. Do you see that? Do you see how your high standards for others have led you to this point in your life?"

You could practically see the steam coming out of William's ears. "All I can see is that the standards in this hospital are not very high. I'm disappointed."

"Do me a favor and think about that while you're here."

Later, Dr. F. told me that in his experience, many patients were admitted to Bullfinch with severe depressive symptoms that had their origins not in a chemical imbalance, but in patterns of behavior that they had learned since they were young. In William's case, he had developed "narcissistic traits," meaning that he enhanced his self-esteem by criticizing other people. Sometimes, this tactic worked, but eventually, it led to rejection and depression. The best treatment, he believed, was long-term psychotherapy, though medications were appropriate to treat severe psychiatric symptoms when they flared up.

William stayed on the unit for about a week. The day after his interview with Dr. F., he seemed much calmer and no longer the entitled and aggressive person that he appeared to be when he was first admitted. I doubted that this transformation was purely due to Dr. F.'s intervention, since William was also taking strong tranquilizing medications. He ceased reminding me of my low position on the Harvard totem pole, and we had a couple of interesting conversations. We talked about what he should say to his girlfriend about why he was admitted to a psychiatric hospital. He decided to tell her the truth. When I swung by his room sometime later to find out how that conversation went, he told me that she said that the relationship was over.

His response was telling. At first, he behaved as one might predict in a patient with narcissistic personality disorder. He was blasé, and told me that it was high time they broke up anyway. He complained that she had been "getting on my nerves," and he looked forward to moving on. But the next day, I learned from the nurses that he had a long tearful conversation with her later that night. When I met with him, he said that he had realized how much she meant to him, and had pleaded with her to try to work things out. She agreed to make the effort.

I praised him.

"That's great," I said. "But what about what you told me yesterday, how annoying she was. Was that true? Or were you saying that just to protect yourself from the pain of being rejected?"

"Aren't you quite the psychiatrist?" he said. "I see you've been taking lessons from your superiors."

But he didn't look particularly angry or mocking when he said this. It seemed almost a reflexive response. Playing into his narcissism, I said, "Yes, I can certainly use all the help I can get at this stage in the game. But you haven't answered my question."

"Sure, okay," he said with a smirk, "I was putting up a bit of a shield to 'protect' myself."

"I know sarcasm when I hear it."

"No, I'm telling you the truth. I'm willing to learn from my errors. Anybody who wants to excel has to be willing to take constructive criticism. I've always been at the top of my profession, and if my consultants give me some good advice, I'm willing to take it. That also applies to Dr. F. and any of his underlings. *I* didn't go to medical school."

I had to admire William's ability to reframe every situation in order to coincide with his exalted self-image. The idea that his psychiatrists might be in charge of his care was intolerable to him, so he simply redefined us as his "consultants." This was his way of coming to terms with the fact that he had problems and needed help.

For me, it was a lesson in the importance of combining medication and psychotherapy. In William's agitated state when he was admitted, he needed something chemical to bring him to a point of being able to look at himself and his behavior patterns objectively. But he needed a lot more than medication to learn certain lessons, for example, that intimacy is crucial, and that humans are more than interchangeable cogs in his life. As I said good-bye to him on his discharge day, I suspected that this was a lesson he would have to encounter several more times before truly learning it.

Dr. F. was willing to use medications when needed, but in his heart of hearts, he believed that the more profound healing took place as a result of psychotherapy. Medicine was a way of "softening up" patients to get them to a point where they could be receptive to therapy. Ingeborg Van Pelt, a pediatrician and headache specialist with an interest in therapy, wrote recently that she uses the following metaphor when she talks to her patients: "Tranquilizers and psychotropic drugs serve as a life jacket—they keep you afloat, but they do not show you the way back to shore."[5] Therapy gets patients back to shore.

But powerful MGH faculty members disagreed with this prioritizing of therapy over medication. One afternoon, I went to a department party at the chief resident's house. The Tall Ships had come to Boston, as they did every decade or so, and the department had organized this event to welcome the new residents as we watched these vintage triple-mast boats sail into the Boston harbor.

On the deck, I found myself standing next to Dr. S., a renowned researcher in antidepressants. We had recently admitted one of his patients, Margaret, to Bullfinch 3 for depression. Margaret was young, in her midtwenties, came from a middle-class family, and had no obvious reason to be depressed. Nonetheless, since her sophomore year in college, she had landed in one psychiatric hospital after another. When she became depressed, she was overcome by loneliness, and turned to cutting her arms, not deeply enough to cause dangerous blood loss, but enough to cause pain and scarring. Paradoxically, she saw this as a way of preventing suicide, telling me once that her emotional pain was so intense, it actually felt like a relief to cut herself. By transforming the emotional pain into something physical, it distracted her from her depression.

Once she was on the unit, Dr. F. had evaluated her and diagnosed her with borderline personality disorder, which refers to a lifelong pattern of emptiness and desperate attempts to get other people to fill the emotional gap.[6] Such patients find themselves unable to cope with rejection and do impulsive things to quickly change their mood state, such as drinking, using drugs, striking out at others, or superficial cutting. Nobody knows how the disorder develops, but having been abused by one's parents, either physically or sexually, seems to be a risk factor. Looking through the notes from prior hospitalizations in her chart, it was clear that many caregivers had suspected a history of sexual abuse, but Margaret had consistently denied it.

Dr. S. had tried Margaret on various medications over the years, many of which seemed to help for a period of months, but inevitably her moods would worsen eventually, and she would be hospitalized. Dr. F., looking over her long list of medications, commented with his usual bluntness during morning rounds, "This woman is borderline, that's her problem. You can do anything you want with her meds but it isn't going to make a difference unless she gets into therapy." In fact, she was seeing a therapist, but often standard psychodynamic therapy did not work for borderline personality disorder, and a new approach, called dialectical behavior therapy, known by its initials as DBT, looked promising in clinical trials.[7] Dr. F. thought a referral to a DBT therapist was more important than a new antidepressant cocktail.

When I told Dr. S. about Dr. F.'s take on his patient, he shook his head, irritated. "Looking at someone with that degree of depression and talking about borderline personality is like coming here to look at the tall ships but then focusing on the dinghies. Therapy won't work until you treat the underlying biological syndrome." For Dr. S., a far bigger challenge was to get patients to agree to take antidepressants, which they were often reluctant to continue because of the stigma attached to being on psych meds. "You have only one life to live, you don't want to live it depressed," he would tell them. His point was that anyone with a depression of her severity would become irritable and impulsively self-destructive, behaving in ways that mimic borderline personality disorder. But he had observed that once the depression was adequately treated, such "personality disorders" would melt away. Margaret spent a week and a half at Bullfinch and improved modestly with a combination of all the things we provided—medication adjustments, intensive daily individual and group therapy, a safe place, bland but reliable hospital meals, crafts, etc. . . . She was discharged when we felt she was unlikely to harm herself at home.

Who was right about Margaret's underlying problem—Dr. F. or Dr. S.? There is still no way of knowing. While the debate about the origins of mental illness remained unresolved, many of the MGH faculty nevertheless gravitated to opposite polls of the biology-versus-environment divide, based apparently on the kinds of treatment techniques they preferred. The psychodynamic psychiatrists loved doing psychotherapy, believing that its benefits were more profound and long lasting. The biological psychiatrists were taken with the logical process of prescribing medications, having seen many successes in their patients.[8]

Debates aside, the main thing that you learn in a psychiatric residency, then or now, is how to write prescriptions. Thus, during my inpatient rotations I ordered long lists of medications in the nurse's order book; I ordered tranquilizers and antipsychotics for patients who flooded into the psychiatric emergency room; and I wrote prescriptions for experimental combinations of antidepressants and mood stabilizers in the psychopharmacology clinic, where all the clinical research took place.

To the layperson, psychopharmacology seems complicated, because there are dozens of different medications to keep track of, frequent Food and Drug Administration announcements about new indications, and long lists of drug interactions and side effects. For patients who do not respond well to the first few medications we try, coming up with the right cocktail is, indeed, sometimes perplexing and requires a sophisticated and highly experienced prescriber. In most cases, however, the drugs we prescribe consist of "me-too" versions of one original medication.

In any profession, tricks of the trade make complex information manageable, and the trick in psychopharmacology is to realize that there are only a handful of umbrella categories of psychotropic drugs. Once you memorize the properties of these categories, you have also memorized the characteristics of the many drugs within each class. The clinical work involves talking to a patient and looking for a pattern of symptoms that matches up to a medication's profile of effectiveness. Once you've decided on a category such as the SSRIs, choosing, say, Zoloft over Celexa is a combination of guesswork and personal preference. In making the decision, we might consider whether someone in the patient's family has responded to a given drug, whether there are particular side effects we want to avoid, or whether the patient strongly requests a certain agent, commonly in response to a TV commercial.

Learning how to do therapy was, by comparison, a complicated and mysterious endeavor. It was like sailing without a compass. The lectures taught us the theory, but in order to learn the skills we were simply thrown into a room with a patient. After muddling through the hour, we met with supervisors to discuss our cases. Working from detailed notes, we would recapitulate what happened in each session, and the supervisor would tell us what we did right or wrong.

At first, I felt like an imposter as I escorted new patients from the crowded clinic waiting room into an office. "I'm Dr. Carlat," I would say. "What brought you to the clinic today?" The patients, assuming that I was a legitimate and well-trained therapist, would open the floodgates and tell me everything. I learned quickly that one of the crucial skills required for therapy is the ability to shut up and listen.

For example, one of my first therapy patients during residency was a woman in her thirties who came in because she was worried about her job. She was a sleekly dressed, portfolio-carrying businesswoman. We sat down in the office, and she immediately unleashed a torrent of emotion, speaking angrily and tearfully about her unreasonable boss, her annoying coworkers, and her conviction that she was about to get fired. Her transformation from a high-powered executive to an overwrought patient with streaming mascara was all the more remarkable because: (a) I was an utter stranger; and (b) Other than a few strategically placed utterances like "Uh huh" and "Go on," I said almost nothing. Nonetheless, at the end of the session she took a big breath and said, "Thank you, this has been so helpful." Sometimes, therapy was part catharsis, part confession, and required little skill beyond listening empathically.

Usually, however, being a good therapist entails more than being a friendly sounding board. Most of my patients would take a few minutes to outline the gist of their predicament, pause, and then look expectantly at me. This was my cue to say something profound or to ask a question that might cut to the core of their issues. I was often at a loss. During my post-session supervision, the most urgent question I had for my supervisors was, "What do I say next?" In essence, this is the key skill of therapy—knowing what to say, or what *not* to say, next.

Supervisors told me to ask the patient, "Why *now*?" Life problems rarely emerge fully formed on the day of a first therapy appointment. They have been developing and festering over the course of many years. Why did the patient choose to call the therapy clinic and to book an appointment on the particular day they did? This, presumably, would provide a clue to the crux of the issue.

Virginia, for example, was a twenty-five-year-old woman with panic disorder. In response to my "why *now*" question, she said she called after her boyfriend canceled a date, saying he wanted to go out with his friends to watch a baseball game. Her core issue turned out to be a fear of relationships, because she believed they inevitably led to rejection. Another patient, Jim, a thirty-one-year-old graduate student, called after receiving a poor grade on a paper he had turned in. He was overcome with anger and disgust with his professor. His core issue, predictably, was difficulty dealing with authority figures, beginning with his father.

Eventually, my patients would have presented the basic problems, and this was where the real therapeutic "work" was supposed to begin. At that point, as a neophyte therapist, I would really panic, since there is no single recipe for effective therapy. While research shows that just about all therapies *work*, studies have been unable to show any clear advantages of one technique over the others. There are three basic kinds of therapy: "supportive" therapy, in which you listen sympathetically and provide commonsense advice; "psychodynamic" therapy, in which you dig into the past and show patients how dysfunctional early family relationships seep into the present; and finally, cognitive behavioral therapy, a problem-solving approach in which you identify a patient's self-defeating thoughts, trace how the thoughts are affecting his or her emotions and behaviors, and then work on revising these thoughts. A farcical version of this technique was made famous on *Saturday Night Live* by Al Franken's "therapist" character Stuart Smalley, who admonished patients: "That's just stinkin' thinkin'."

Most of my supervisors specialized in psychodynamic therapy, probably because they had done their training during a time when Freudian psychoanalytic theory was dominant. My psychodynamic supervisors wanted me to pay plenty of attention to the unconscious motivations of patients, which often were thought to have sexual undertones. Like most other residents, I was skeptical of the idea that unlocking repressed sexuality was the key to psychological health, but I got a chance to test the theory with one of my first therapy patients.

Brenda was a young graduate student who was struggling with her relationship with her boyfriend, who she said was not attentive enough. "He just doesn't do the things boyfriends are supposed to do," she said, "like buying me flowers when I do well on an exam, or taking me out to dinner." Although Brenda was technically beautiful, with her dark hair, blue eyes, and small features, she carried herself stiffly and rarely smiled. When I told my supervisor, Dr. M., about our first meeting, she wondered about how Brenda made *me* feel. Was I attracted to her? It seemed an uncomfortable topic, but I admitted that I was, indeed, attracted to her physically, but that her icy demeanor put me off.

"That's very important data for your therapy with Brenda," said Dr. M. "Because however she makes you feel is likely how she is making other people in her life feel."

"Like her boyfriend?"

She nodded. "Her boyfriend, her family, her friends. Patients re-create situations in the office that they are familiar with outside of the office. Your job is to use your relationship with Brenda as a way of putting up a mirror, so that she can learn what she does in her important relationships outside of therapy."

That made sense. In fact, it sounded like an intriguing and powerful way to help people change. If it worked, that is.

Unfortunately, over the year that I spent doing weekly sessions with Brenda, I had a very hard time lifting up that mirror with any skill. Our sessions would begin promisingly. Brenda started by bringing me up to date on her life, telling me a story about the latest failing of her boyfriend, for instance. But I had a hard time knowing where to go next. I heard myself asking those annoyingly shrinky questions, like "And how did you feel about that?" Or I would make empathic statements like "You must have felt angry when he did that." She would agree that she did feel angry, but we couldn't seem to get deeper. When I tried to make connections with her relationship with her father, she didn't agree or just didn't have much to add. I began to sense a tension in the room. I assumed that she saw me as a useless therapist, and I saw her as a stiff patient who was stingy with her words.

"Now you know exactly how her boyfriend feels," said Dr. M. "Comment on that in the next session."

That struck me as an awkward thing to bring up, but I tried.

"Brenda, I detect tension. You seem to be frustrated or unhappy with me. I wonder if this is the same kind of tension that comes up between you and your boyfriend?"

She frowned and looked away. "No, I don't think so. I'm just not sure we are making much progress in therapy."

I recounted the session to Dr. M. "You went too quickly with your interpretation," she commented. "You should have just brought up the tension and not tried to connect it to her boyfriend. That was too threatening for her at this stage in the treatment."

Her case ended up somewhat disastrously from my perspective. She abruptly told me one day that she was going to look for a different therapist. Knowing that Dr. M. would want me to schedule a session or two for proper closure, I suggested this to Brenda. She bristled, saying, "I don't think so." In fact, she couldn't get out of the office quickly enough, leaving halfway through our allotted time.

In processing it, Dr. M. thought that Brenda was not ready to tangle with the important issues. I was less sure. I wondered if I was just a bad therapist, or if the psychodynamic technique didn't work as well as it was supposed to. More than anything else, it made me realize how difficult and imprecise is the entire process of therapy, whether you are therapist or patient.

Meanwhile, across campus in the Warren Building, the biological psychiatrist George Murray had had it up to here with therapy. "Why do psychiatrists dick around with chickenshit?" he challenged us. Therapy, he said, too often devolved into "psychosocial taffy," "holistic fajaba" (his made-up term), or "chronic undifferentiated psychotherapy."

George Murray was an attending on the psychiatric consult-liaison service, a troupe of psychiatrists who were on call to the medical and surgical wards in case a medically ill patient needed urgent psychiatric attention. Examples included postsurgical patients who became delirious and violent because of a bad reaction to pain meds and antibiotics, patients who had made serious suicide attempts and were recovering from self-inflicted gunshot wounds or falls out of windows, and those who wanted to leave the hospital against medical advice. We visited these patients with the attendings, one of whom was George Murray.

Because the consult-liaison faculty was constantly dealing with medical issues, they were particularly prone to see psychiatry as a medical rather than a psychological specialty. They approached mental illness as though it were a brain disease, and they focused on a complicated brain circuit called the "limbic system," which Murray called the "playground of psychiatry." He thought that most symptoms of mental illness, such as anxiety, depression, and rage, could be traced to the limbic system.

According to this theory, mental symptoms arise in the same way patients with epilepsy have seizures. Neurons normally fire in sequence, like a string of firecrackers, but in epilepsy, a brain defect leads to all the firecrackers discharging at once, causing a seizure-induced shaking of the entire body. But sometimes seizure activity is focused in specific areas of the brain, such as the temporal lobe (home to most of the limbic system). In "temporal lobe epilepsy," the neurons ignite themselves in very specific brain centers, causing panic, rage, or depression, depending on the region affected.

Though Murray was the first to admit that there was little solid evidence that limbic seizures actually caused most psychiatric illnesses, he found it a compelling metaphor. And the fact that drugs used to treat epilepsy are sometimes helpful in psychiatry seemed to lend credence to the theory. Depakote and Tegretol are two antiseizure drugs that have proven to be effective for bipolar disorder. But I was never convinced, because we were never able to actually prove that our patients experienced these seizures. For example, we consulted on a man who was recovering from injuries sustained during a car accident. It was a case of road rage, in which the patient was cut off by another driver who gave him the finger, and he accelerated toward him. His car lost control and it rolled over onto the shoulder of the highway. He was now recovering from a fractured vertebra.

In interviewing him, it was clear that he frequently had attacks of rage disproportionate to situations. During a petty argument with his wife, for instance, he threw a plate against a wall, shattering it. Murray thought he had temporal lobe epilepsy, which can cause abrupt rage episodes. We ordered a brain wave test called an EEG, but it was normal. "That means nothing," said Murray. "He might have been between seizures when he had the test." He decided to put him on the anti-epileptic drug Depakote. The man had no rage attacks during his admission, but I didn't know if that was due to the Depakote or the potent mix of narcotics for his pain.

Over time, the enthusiasm for invoking temporal lobe epilepsy as a cause of psychiatric symptoms has begun to fade, because it is so difficult to prove its presence in patients.[9] It has been replaced by a plethora of other theories, mostly revolving around levels of neurotransmitters and hormones. While yet unproven, these biological theories continue to allure psychiatrists and their patients who seek clear answers to the intangible symptoms of mental illness. After I finished my residency, I, like many of my fellow residents, became a psychopharmacologist, focusing on brief fifteen- to twenty-minute medication visits. While I now regret having started my career like this, it was in some ways inevitable that I would have done so. The stars were aligned. Therapy was mysterious, and often frustrating. Prescribing medications was clear-cut, more lucrative, and reinforced my self-image as a "real" doctor. Only later did I realize how crucial are the skills of psychotherapy, even for those whose main practice is prescribing medication.

Chapter 3

The Bible of Psychiatry

Lorraine was twenty-four years old, married, had a promising career—and she was falling apart.

I was interviewing her in my private practice office in Newburyport. I had finished my residency at Mass General a couple of years earlier and had set up shop in a nineteenth-century brick building with a view of a white-steepled church. It had not taken me long to become fairly busy, since there weren't many psychiatrists an hour north of Boston.

"I don't know what's wrong with me," Lorraine said. "I can't seem to do anything. I can't even drive to work."

As she pulled her brown hair behind her ears, she began to cry. I handed her the box of Kleenex that I always keep on my desk.

"I'm on temporary disability," she explained, pulling a tissue from the box. "I can't believe it. I've always worked. I love my job."

This was our first meeting. Lorraine had been referred to me by her primary care doctor, who asked me to treat her for anxiety.

"She seems to have some combination of anxiety and depression," her doctor had told me over the phone. "I gave her some Valium, but I don't think it's helped."

In Newburyport, primary care doctors often try to handle their patients' psychiatric problems rather than waiting the month or two required before their patients can get an appointment with a psychiatrist. Often, that works fine. Internists can prescribe the full range of antidepressants and antianxiety pills, and they get plenty of experience, given how common psychiatric problems are. But in Lorraine's case, her antianxiety drug was not working. My job was to do a structured interview to see if I could discover a diagnosis that was being missed, and then to come up with a more appropriate treatment.

A psychiatric interview has a certain rhythm to it. You start by listening to what your patient says for a few minutes, without interrupting, all the while sorting through possible diagnoses. This vast landscape of distress has been mapped into a series of categories in the DSM,[1] psychiatry's diagnostic manual, now in its fourth edition. The book breaks down mental suffering into sixteen groups of disorders, such as those of mood, anxiety, psychosis, and memory. As I listened to Lorraine, it was clear to me that she had one of the anxiety disorders, but which one? There are twelve options listed among DSM-IV's menu of nearly four hundred psychiatric diagnoses.

I learned that Lorraine was a paralegal, talented and well liked by her employer. But over the last year she had noticed a mounting anxiety every morning as she got ready for her commute. Once on the road, the frightful Boston commuter traffic gave her a sensation of being trapped—to an extent a normal response, but in Lorraine it had become extreme. She had panic attacks daily, during which she felt suddenly claustrophobic and suffocated, captured by an urgent need to get off the highway. Her heart pounded rapidly, she would sweat profusely, she became dizzy and was convinced that she was about to faint, though she never did. She would pull off at the nearest exit, and once her anxiety subsided, she would complete her commute on surface streets.

After she described these symptoms to me, she came right out and asked me a question that I believe is often at the back of patients' minds: "Am I going crazy?"

"No," I said, "you're not going crazy. You're having panic attacks. I see this all the time—let me explain what happens."

I went on to talk to her about how panic attacks start, what sort of symptoms they cause, and how readily they are treated. In doing so, I was taking advantage of one of the best qualities of DSM-IV—its ability to help organize the chaos of experience. In asking me if she was crazy, Lorraine was saying she was overwhelmed by what she was going through. Not only was she having panic attacks, but, in a vicious spiral of mounting anxiety, she was terrified of what these attacks represented. Was she really "losing it"? Would she end up strapped to a bed in a psychiatric ward, requiring injections of sedatives from the modern equivalents of Nurse Ratched from *One Flew over the Cuckoo's Nest*?

DSM assigns each slice of craziness with a name and a number. Panic disorder, for example, is disease number 300.21, a diagnostic code that I must provide to the insurance company to get reimbursed. Naming psychiatric disorders reassures patients, who often improve markedly just by hearing that they have a condition that is well-recognized and treatable. But just because it has a name, is it actually a disease? We commonly think of diseases as collections of symptoms with clear biological origins. Psychiatric diseases are similar but different. They are indeed collections of symptoms, but without any clear biological cause. Because of this, we come up with our diagnoses through the kinds of long conversations that I had with Lorraine.

In order to confirm that she had panic attacks, I asked her about thirteen possible panic symptoms as listed in DSM-IV. Patients must report at least four to qualify, and Lorraine easily met the cut, reporting six: shortness of breath, palpitations, dizziness, sweating, shaking, and a fear of fainting. But having had a panic attack per se doesn't mean you have panic disorder. Panic attacks are common. Being claustrophobic, I've had two panic attacks—once while sitting in the cabin of a hot airplane stuck on the tarmac in Washington, D.C., and once while crawling through the Vietcong tunnels as a tourist in Vietnam.

But in order to be diagnosed with panic disorder, you have to have panic attacks that are so frequent and so severe that they interfere with everyday functioning. The task of a psychiatrist is to understand the definitions of our diseases, and to efficiently ask all the right questions and to interpret the answers appropriately.

"How often do you have these panic attacks?" I asked Lorraine.

"At least once every day during the week."

"What about on the weekends?"

"Only on Sunday night, when I start worrying about having to drive to work the next day. All I can think about is that I might have a panic attack on the road."

"And do you find yourself worrying or thinking about panic attacks much of the time?"

"All the time!"

Clearly, anxiety was taking over Lorraine's life, and the anxiety was somehow triggered by her work life. But why now? She said nothing had changed at work. The panic attacks, she said, seemed to come out of the blue.

In an earlier era, this is where the work of a psychiatrist would really begin. We would dig. We would ask pointed questions. We wouldn't let the patient off the hook until we had figured out what made him or her *tick*.

No longer. The tradition of psychological curiosity has been dying a gradual death, and the DSM is part cause, part consequence of this transformation of our profession. These days, psychiatrists are less interested in "why" and more interested in "what." In the past, when most psychiatrists were psychoanalysts, treatment entailed constructing elaborate explanations for how symptoms developed through early childhood experiences. Anxiety was thought to be caused when the conscious mind came face-to-face with unconscious desires and hidden memories—often of a sexual nature. If Lorraine had seen a psychiatrist in the 1950s or 1960s, chances were good that she would have had dozens of weekly fifty-minute sessions during which a clinician would listen quietly, seeking patterns and themes. The climax of treatment would be an "interpretation," a statement like "You have always been terrified of male attention, beginning with your father—no wonder you are having panic attacks as you walk into the office of your boss, who, like your father, is an all-powerful male who holds your future in his hands."[2]

Many such explanations were, no doubt, true, but unfortunately the truth did not necessarily set patients free. Symptoms stubbornly remained. Gradually, the profession became disillusioned with psychoanalysis, and turned to other methods, such as psychopharmacology. The DSM provided a method that helped us make medication decisions. It is the main tool of what is termed "descriptive psychiatry," in which we paint a detailed picture of the patient's symptoms and try to come up with just the right label to reflect that picture.

Similarly, part of the psychiatric interview is a series of questions designed to rule out syndromes within all the categories of DSM. Thus, after I ascertained that Lorraine indeed had panic disorder, rather than drilling down into the causes of her anxiety, I went on to systematically ask her about syndromes in the other major categories of DSM-IV, including depression, psychosis, eating disorders, dementia, substance abuse, and so on.

I began with depression, because it often accompanies anxiety. There are nine possible DSM-IV symptoms of major depression, and patients who have five of the nine for at least two weeks receive the diagnosis.

"Aside from the anxiety you've been feeling lately," I began, "have you also been feeling down and blue?"

"I'm always sad," she responded, "because I never thought I would have to live this way."

"Has the sadness been so bad that you wish you were dead?"

"No, I'm not suicidal, if that's what you mean. I could never do that to my family."

"I'm glad to hear that. It sounds like you still have hope, then?" (There is a criterion of depression called "hopelessness," which I was getting at here.)

"I have hope. That's why I'm here."

After I asked some more questions, it was clear that Lorraine had four depressive symptoms: sadness, insomnia, poor concentration, and poor energy. But she didn't have the following: suicidality, appetite changes, agitation, lack of the ability to experience pleasure, or hopelessness. Because she had four rather than five out of nine symptoms, she didn't qualify for major depression.

To review: Four out of thirteen panic symptoms equals panic disorder; five of nine depressive symptoms equals depression; and so on through the dozens of other disorders listed in our peculiar bible. Is there something in the human brain that dictates these numbering rules? Of course not. The modern criteria for depression and other diagnoses are human constructions, and were created in 1980 by a committee of the American Psychiatric Association, which ultimately published the DSM-III and defined the criteria for nearly three hundred other psychiatric diseases.

Over the years, the various versions of the DSM have been criticized and ridiculed. The book has been called a tool of the pharmaceutical industry and a collection of arbitrary labels based on shaky science. But with all its imperfections, it actually evolved out of a crying need in the profession for more precise descriptions of disorders, and it has done a great service by providing them. DSM actually represents the culmination of a profession's noble struggle to categorize the inner anarchy that is psychiatric illness.

The story of DSM properly starts in 1890, in Heidelberg, Germany, when a psychiatrist named Emil Kraepelin was hired to run a prominent psychiatric hospital.[3] In the late 1800s, the classification of mental illness was primitive. There were two widely acknowledged categories: "insanity" (which included what we now call schizophrenia, bipolar disorder, and dementia) and "mental deficiency" (which comprised mental retardation and other developmental disorders).

At this time, most psychiatric research was done by neurologists, who studied slices of brain tissue in search of the presumed defects responsible for mental illness. To quote the historian Edward Shorter, the late 1800s saw an "absolute craze for studying psychiatry with microscopes." There was reason behind this craze, because by then psychiatrists had already discovered the cause of one version of insanity—neurosyphilis.

Since the late 1700s, physicians had described people who would suddenly behave bizarrely several years after having caught syphilis through sexual contact. We now know that the microorganisms, or "spirochetes," that cause syphilis go quiescent after causing transient genital sores. Decades may elapse before the spirochetes invade the brain, eventually causing psychiatric and neurological symptoms. Sometimes, the very first symptoms of neurosyphilis looked very much like mania. For example, according to Shorter's *A History of Psychiatry*, a distinguished mid-nineteenth-century German chemistry professor once "suddenly interrupted his lecture and started to tell gossipy stories from the city. The previous day he had gone out and bought 10 automobiles and 100 wristwatches." The sudden onset of mania in a middle-aged male was considered to be neurosyphilis unless proven otherwise. Unfortunately, the illness was generally fatal until the advent of penicillin in the 1940s.

For Kraepelin, neurosyphilis, which was sometimes called "general paresis of the insane," provided a clear model of a form of insanity with an identifiable neuropathological explanation. It stood to reason that other forms of insanity would also yield their secrets to the microscope.

Assuming that all mental illnesses were discrete diseases with yet-to-be-discovered biological roots, Kraepelin decided that a first step in disentangling the causes was to more accurately classify the diseases. He developed a simple but effective method. Every time a patient was admitted to his hospital, he pulled out a card and wrote down the patient's name and presumed diagnosis. He would observe them and note highlights of their symptoms. When they were discharged, he wrote down the final diagnosis. He amassed hundreds of diagnostic cards, and spent his weekends looking for patterns. Which patients got better, and which patients stayed the same or worsened?

What Kraepelin discovered electrified the world of psychiatry. Rather than there being a single category called insanity, Kraepelin found that this label combined two very different types of patients. First, there were patients who became psychotic when young (in their teens or early twenties), and who generally never recovered. He called this disorder *dementia praecox*, Latin for "premature dementia." Later, Eugen Bleuler, a Swiss psychiatrist, renamed this disorder "schizophrenia," from the Greek for "split mind."

Kraepelin's second group of patients became ill somewhat later in life, had episodes of depression or mania (with or without psychosis), and, unlike the first group, tended to recover. He labeled these patients "manic-depressive." Today, we would say that some of these patients had bipolar disorder, which is a condition of alternating depression and mania, while some had "unipolar" depression, that is, depression without manic episodes.

Kraepelin's discovery revolutionized psychiatry because it gave clinicians a way of predicting the course and prognosis of patients. If Kraepelin's new diagnostic scheme suggested that a given patient had dementia praecox (schizophrenia), he could inform the patient's family that the illness was dire, was unlikely to improve much, and might well last for decades. However, if a patient had Kraepelin's "manic depression," he could provide the good news that the patient would improve and might well behave normally for long stretches between episodes of depression or mania.

Unfortunately, aside from defining the outcomes, Kraepelin could do little else, because there were no effective treatments in his day. Patients were housed in asylums, where conditions varied from chaos and bedlam (in fact, the very word "bedlam" was derived from the name of one of the oldest asylums, Bethlem of London) to the relatively well-run and clean asylums in nineteenth-century Germany. A major component of "treatment" was the use of restraints to keep patients from harming themselves, but over time, some symptomatic treatments were developed and used. In the 1800s, for example, psychiatrists often prescribed extremely high dosages of laxatives, under the theory that the diarrhea and catharsis they induced would cut short the more severe psychotic episodes. Morphine injections enjoyed a burst of popularity in asylums for several decades. The drug worked well as a sedative and as a temporary mood elevator, but eventually doctors discovered how addictive it was and ceased its routine use. Other sedatives, such as chloral hydrate and "bromides," were used at various times and were symptomatically helpful, but were hardly cures. The sad fact is that before modern pharmaceuticals, mentally ill people lived their lives often confined to squalid wards, and were at the mercy of their hallucinations, agitated manic spells, and suicidal depressions.

Kraepelin, by systematically categorizing insanity, kick-started the process of searching for biologically based treatments. But had Kraepelin discovered real diseases? He assumed that he had. He believed that if a group of patients shared the same course and prognosis, chances were good that they shared the same biological cause. While acknowledging that psychiatric science was too primitive to identify the actual brain defects causing these illnesses, he hoped that he had succeeded in discovering actual disease entities, thereby "carving nature at its joints." He had laid out the basic buckets of symptoms. He hoped that, over time, science would fill the buckets with more and more biological knowledge, so that, for example, manic depression would be understood just as biologically as endocrinologists now understand the symptoms of diabetes.

Fast forward to December 2007. It was a sunny but chilly winter day in Irvington, a leafy suburb a short subway ride north of Manhattan. I was standing in front of the home of Robert Spitzer, the modern-day Emil Kraepelin, a man who has become a living legend because he has almost single-handedly created the vocabulary of modern psychiatry. I rang the doorbell, and the door swung open. Facing me was Spitzer, wearing an apron, holding a spatula, and smiling as he asked me a distinctly nonpsychiatric question: "Hi. How would you like your eggs?"

"Scrambled," I replied, and we shook hands. I had e-mailed Spitzer a month earlier requesting an interview, and he had taken me up on my offer, inviting me to his home for breakfast and for conversation about his favorite topic—DSM.

Spitzer was elderly but not frail. I noticed a slight tremor of his hands and a limp in his gait, but his white-bearded face appeared vital, and he was still sharp enough to debate the fine points of psychiatric diagnosis, a skill that had gained him international fame.

In the 1970s, Spitzer[4] was a young professor of psychiatry at Columbia University, and he had been tangentially involved in helping to write the second version of DSM—DSM-II,[5] which had been published in 1968 (the very first DSM had been published in 1952). The DSM-II had been a small spiral-bound manual, a little over one hundred pages listing 182 diagnoses. Its descriptions of disorders were vague and often referred to the concept of "neurosis," a term from psychoanalysis that has essentially disappeared from modern psychiatry. For example, in DSM-II, depression was referred to as "depressive neurosis" and was defined in a single sentence: "This disorder is manifested by an excessive reaction of depression due to an internal conflict or to an identifiable event such as the loss of a love object or cherished possession."

Given such brief and vague definitions, psychiatrists would often disagree on how to apply diagnoses to particular patients. The technical term for this problem is "poor diagnostic reliability." Studies done in the 1950s and 1960s found that the rates of diagnostic agreement between psychiatrists when faced with the same patient were embarrassingly low, from 32 percent to 42 percent.[6] How much confidence could you have in your doctor if it was likely a psychiatrist across town would give you a completely different diagnosis?

The American Psychiatric Association, impressed with Spitzer's grasp of diagnostic categories, hired him in 1974 to oversee the creation of DSM-III, a newer version of DSM, which would help to solve the reliability problem. Spitzer and his colleagues reworked the manual in order to make the definitions of disorders more specific and objective. In their new system, each diagnosis was defined by a list of symptoms, each of which was described in enough detail to ensure that any psychiatrist would recognize their presence. They then defined a numerical threshold for each diagnosis, and if a patient met the minimum threshold number of symptoms, he or she "qualified" for the diagnosis.

In addition to beefing up the definitions of existing disorders, the committee added more disorders, so that the book increased in girth from 100 pages to 494 pages, and from 182 diagnoses to 265. Some of the new diagnoses included borderline personality disorder, narcissistic personality disorder, post-traumatic stress disorder, and social anxiety disorder. In some cases, they deleted diagnoses that reflected outdated cultural mores and were controversial. For example, in DSM-II, homosexuality was considered a mental disorder, described as a "sexual deviation," and categorized in the same section as pedophilia. In DSM-III, homosexuality per se was no longer considered a disease; instead, there was a new syndrome called "ego-dystonic homosexuality," reserved for people whose homosexuality had caused them to become depressed.

I asked Spitzer how all these decisions about adding or deleting diagnoses were made.

"Ultimately," he said, "they were made by votes of a committee. We started with the categories that were already listed in DSM-II, and we brainstormed about other disorders that were being discussed in the psychiatric literature but which had not yet been formally defined."

"And how did you decide on the specific symptoms that would qualify a patient for a diagnosis?"

"There was a group of psychiatrists at Washington University in St. Louis who had already been working on what were called 'research diagnostic criteria.' This was an early effort to create reliable diagnoses for clinical research, and we based some of our diagnoses on these."[7]

"But ultimately, was it just a committee decision?" I asked, thinking about my patient Lorraine, who just missed the depression diagnosis. "I mean, how did you decide, for example, on *five* criteria as being your minimum threshold for depression?"

"It was just a consensus," he said. "We would ask clinicians and researchers, 'How many symptoms do you think patients ought to have before you would give the diagnosis of depression?' And we came up with the arbitrary number of five."

"But why did you choose five and not four? Or why didn't you choose six?" I persisted.

He smiled impishly, saying, "Because four just seemed like not enough. And six seemed like too much."

"But weren't there any studies done to establish the threshold?"

"We did reviews of the literature, and in some cases we received funding from NIMH to do field trials."

In field trials, psychiatrists were recruited to "test-drive" proposed criteria. Typically, they would be asked to diagnose patients with depression (or other disorders) according to their best clinical judgment. Then, they would be given a long list of proposed DSM-III criteria, and asked to check off those which the patient met. The committee would look at this data to determine which of the criteria were deemed most important by practicing psychiatrists. They would estimate the minimum threshold of criteria from this data. This was tricky, and required quite a bit of judgment on the part of the committee. If you set the threshold too low, then too many people with only modest symptoms would get diagnosed; but if you set it too high, there was a risk of missing genuinely ill people who needed treatment.

When pressed, Spitzer admitted that even with the information from this research, arbitrary decisions had to be made.

"When you do field trials in depression and other disorders, there is no sharp dividing line where you can confidently say, 'This is the perfect number of symptoms needed to make a diagnosis.' With increasing numbers of symptoms you get increasing disability, and increased suffering, but there is no sharp cutoff point. It would be nice if we had a biological gold standard, which you could correlate with the number of symptoms, but that doesn't exist, because we don't understand the neurobiology of depression."

As Spitzer spoke, I was reminded of Emil Kraepelin, who was faced with precisely the same quandary. He single-handedly performed his own rudimentary versions of the DSM field trials, in which he correlated patients' symptoms with how psychiatrically impaired they became. He was able to distinguish broad categories of pathology, hoping that psychiatrists in a hundred years would finally discover the biological markers for these diseases. But the brain is far too complex, and psychiatric diagnosis remains as much art as science.

As for depression, so it went for all the other psychiatric disorders. Spitzer and his group of experts met, discussed the scientific literature, looked at the field trial data, added a sprinkling of clinical wisdom, and voted on criteria for diagnosing schizophrenia, bipolar disorder, panic disorder, and nearly three hundred other sources of suffering.

After DSM-III came DSM-III-R (for "revised") in 1987, then DSM-IV in 1994, and DSM-IV-TR ("text revised") in 2000. With each subsequent edition, the number of diagnostic categories multiplied, and the books became larger and more expensive. Each became a best seller for the APA, and DSM is now one of the major sources of income for the organization.

But as its popularity among clinicians soared, it began to attract a host of critics. For example, the sociologists Herb Kutchins and Stuart Kirk have written two books critical of the DSM and have argued that "DSM is a book of tentatively assembled agreements."[8] DSM, they charged, was capable of finding a diagnosis for everybody. "Where you thought your friends were just having normal troubles," they wrote in their 1997 book *Making Us Crazy*, "the developers of the American Psychiatric Association's diagnostic bible raise the possibility that you are surrounded by the mentally ill. Equally disconcerting to you, you may be among them."[9]

Even the leaders in psychiatry were poking fun at DSM. "The problem is that the diagnostic manual we are using in psychiatry is like a field guide and it just keeps expanding and expanding," noted

Dr. Paul McHugh, a professor of psychiatry at Johns Hopkins University, as quoted in a *New York Times* article. "Pretty soon," he joked, "we'll have a syndrome for short, fat Irish guys with a Boston accent, and I'll be mentally ill."[10]

The most controversial diagnoses are those that define conditions that are sometimes hard to distinguish from normality. For example, Christopher Lane, a literature professor at Northwestern University, has singled out one diagnosis, "social phobia" (sometimes known as "social anxiety disorder"), for particular scorn. DSM-IV defines the disorder thusly:

> A. A persistent fear of one or more social or performance situations in which the person is exposed to unfamiliar people or to possible scrutiny by others.
> B. Exposure to the feared situation almost invariably provokes anxiety, which may take the form of a situationally bound or situationally pre-disposed Panic Attack.
> C. The person recognizes that this fear is unreasonable or excessive.
> D. The feared situations are avoided or else are endured with intense anxiety and distress.[11]

According to Lane, another word for what is being clinically described here is "shyness," which is also the title of his book about the deficiencies of the DSM system.[12] Lane argues that psychiatry has redefined shyness as a disorder, whereas it was once an admired quality, associated with "bookishness, reserve, and a yen for solitude."[13] In his view, psychiatrists like Spitzer took a normal human emotion, met behind closed doors in committees, and transformed it into a disease.

A similar critique has been leveled against PMDD, or "premenstrual dysphoric disorder." Again, paraphrasing DSM-IV, here are the diagnostic criteria:

> In most menstrual cycles during the past year, the following symptoms occur during the week before menstruation: depression, anxiety, mood swings, and lack of interest in activities once enjoyed. The symptoms must be severe enough to markedly interfere with work, school, or usual activities, and they must completely disappear for at least one full week after menstruation.[14]

Like social anxiety disorder, PMDD's symptoms sound very much like a "condition" that is a normal part of life. In its less severe form, this is premenstrual disorder, or PMS, and affects about 85 percent of all women. In an article called "The Strange Case of Dr. Jekyll and Ms. Hyde: How PMS Became a Cultural Phenomenon and a Psychiatric Disorder," Joan Chrisler and Paula Caplan argue that PMDD is an illusory label for normal discomfort.[15] "Women are supposed to be cheerleaders," commented one of the authors. "When a woman is anything but that, she and her family are quick to think something is wrong."[16]

Both social phobia and PMDD point out a troubling vulnerability of most psychiatric diagnoses, which is that they exist on a spectrum. Shyness and menstrual discomfort are normal aspects of experience, and each of these experiences can range from mild to severe. Psychiatrists have cordoned off the most painful versions of normal life, defined them as syndromes, and have given them medical-sounding names. Kutchins and Kirk charge that this leads to the "pathologizing of everyday behaviors."

But I have a problem with these critiques. Although DSM reads like a cookbook, in fact real-life psychiatrists rarely use it as one. We don't read off the list of symptoms to our patients as written in the manual, checking them off in order to mechanically apply a diagnosis. Instead, we ask about the symptoms in the context of both our patients' lives and the larger culture. Some patients might formally qualify for a diagnosis like social phobia, yet have symptoms that are so mild that we would not bother to diagnose or treat them. In fact, most of these patients would never even appear at our door.

On the other hand, there are some patients for whom extreme shyness can become a devastating illness, much worse than Lane's characterization of these people as simply bashful or bookish. For example, one of my colleagues referred a seventeen-year-old patient, Randall, to me for treatment of anxiety. When Randall came into my office, the most striking thing about him was that he could barely look at me. He kept his eyes focused on his lap, and spoke so softly I had to pull my chair closer to hear him.

Randall told me that he hated going to classes, and had skipped so many that he was in danger of failing. He avoided school because he was terrified of social encounters. "When I approach other kids," he said, "I have this overpowering sense of extreme worry." He thought other students were scrutinizing him, ridiculing him for being overweight. He was not paranoid or psychotic—he denied hearing voices or believing that others had malevolent intentions. He was just painfully, excruciatingly shy.

His symptoms perfectly fit the DSM-IV description of "social phobia": "a persistent fear of one or more social or performance situations in which the person is exposed to unfamiliar people or to possible scrutiny by others." I started him on the standard medication treatment for this condition—an SSRI (in his case, Zoloft) and a tranquilizer (Xanax). Randall gradually improved, to the point that he was able to graduate and go on to college. The last time I saw him, he was planning to go on job interviews, social situations that "I wouldn't have been able to even fathom" before his treatment. There has been no transformation in his personality—he still comes into my office appearing shy. He will always be "bookish and reserved," in Lane's terminology. But treatment is allowing him to have a life.

The situation is similar with premenstrual dysphoric disorder. In my experience, patients who actually receive the diagnosis are not simply women who are annoyed and uncomfortable with their PMS. Instead, they are at the end of their rope with their symptoms. Judy, for example, is a patient whom I was already treating for depression. Several months after I first met her, she told me that her depression worsened predictably during the week before her periods. "I feel so uncomfortable in my body," she recounted. "Nothing feels right, I can't even look at my children without screaming at them, and then I start crying. But once I get my period, I feel like I've become a normal person again."

Judy was already taking Prozac at a dose of 20 mg/day. Some studies have shown that simply bumping up the dose of an SSRI during "PMS week" solves the problem of PMDD, and I recommended that she increase her dose to 30 mg of Prozac one week every month, allowing her to avoid the worst of the PMDD symptoms. It worked for her.

Both of these patients illustrate that while the diagnostic labels may sound spurious, there are plenty of people out there who are genuinely suffering from the conditions they describe. As a rule, psychiatrists are not beating the bushes, hungry for new patients, trying to hang a label on perfectly healthy people to drum up business. In fact, the reverse is true. It is the patients who are looking for psychiatrists and often waiting months for an appointment.

This is not to say that there are no problems with DSM—but it is important to be clear about what its deficiencies actually are. By and large, DSM has not created pathology where it does not exist. But it has done something almost as harmful. It has drained the color out of the way we understand and treat our patients. It has deemphasized psychological-mindedness, and replaced it with the illusion that we understand our patients when all we are doing is assigning them labels.

What do I mean? In preparation for this chapter, I leafed through Lorraine's chart (she is the patient who was having panic attacks at work), and realized that over the course of her treatment I had diagnosed her with seven separate diseases: panic disorder, major depression NOS (not otherwise specified), agoraphobia, obsessive compulsive disorder, generalized anxiety disorder, social phobia, and attention deficit disorder.

First, I diagnosed her with panic disorder, then quickly added "agoraphobia," which often accompanies panic disorder (agoraphobia is a fear of having a panic attack in certain places where a quick escape would be difficult). With treatment the panic subsided, but then she began to worry about whether she had left her stove on or her door unlocked—symptoms of obsessive compulsive disorder. Eventually, these symptoms went into quiescence, but then she developed a fear of being seen in public, leading to the diagnosis of social phobia. And so it continued, until Lorraine had racked up quite a list of labels.

The technical term for giving patients multiple different diagnoses, as I did with Lorraine, is "comorbidity," and it has become a widely acknowledged problem of the DSM system. Lorraine didn't actually have seven separate diseases, but because DSM categories often share many symptoms, it is common for patients to appear to qualify for separate disorders. Many psychiatric symptoms are nonspecific, meaning that they appear in the recipe list of many different diagnoses. Difficulty concentrating, for example, is a component of sixteen separate disorders, ranging from problems as diverse as dementia, schizophrenia, bipolar disorder, and ADHD. Insomnia shows up in dozens of disorders, as do impulsivity and changes in appetite.

All this overlap undermines our confidence that DSM's disorders are distinct from one another, and if they are not distinct, then perhaps they are not "real." My sense is that Lorraine, like many of my patients, has some basic underlying vulnerability to anxiety and depression, a vulnerability that probably has some yet-to-be-discovered basis in neurobiology. This underlying "mystery defect" can lead to a multiplicity of symptoms that wax and wane, and DSM allows us to apply different labels to these shifting symptom patterns.

If applying many different labels to patients actually helped us decide on the right treatment, the exercise would be worthwhile. But as it turns out, the precise label often has no effect on which medication I choose. For example, SSRIs like Zoloft are effective for at least a dozen supposedly distinct problems, including depression, panic disorder, OCD, bulimia, post-traumatic stress disorder, hypochondriasis, and so on. The nonspecificity of treatment further undermines our confidence that we understand the true nature of what we are treating.

With Lorraine, I had fallen into the trap of what I call "DSM-think," in which I spent too much time trying to fit her into categories and too little time trying to understand her as a person. This is a common failing of DSM, and one which even Michael First, the editor of DSM-IV, acknowledges. "DSM boils down the complexity of psychiatric disorders," First told me during a lunch interview near his office at Columbia University in New York, where he is a professor of clinical psychiatry. "People who are inclined to want to look for the easiest and the most efficient way to get their work done just grasp onto it, and a huge amount is lost when they do that. We used to joke that DSM should come with a combination lock and you can only open the book if you agree to really explore what is going on in the patient's mind."

DSM, First maintains, is a convenient tool for helping us to describe patients and make treatment decisions, but was never meant to substitute for understanding our patients as people. My friend and colleague Brian Greenfield, a psychiatrist in Montreal, has a similar view.

"For me," he said, "DSM is like a GPS system. It allows me to find the basic location of my patient, so that I can figure out where he is. But once I've found him, I try to put the DSM aside, and I say, 'Brian, wait a minute—are you really communicating with him, are you really making his journey easier?' At that moment, DSM is very far away from me."

All of these deficiencies of the DSM have not gone unnoticed by the leadership of the APA. In 1999, the APA and NIMH began a series of conferences with leading experts to take a close look at DSM with the aim of coming up with a better manual, which will eventually be DSM-V. These meetings became the basis for a 2002 book, *A Research Agenda for DSM-V*.[17]

The *Research Agenda* introduced a term that has come back to haunt the DSM-V committee: "paradigm shift." Acknowledging that we know too little about the true nature of the DSM-IV disorders, the authors argued that DSM-V needed to be much more than just a more refined list of diseases. In their words: "All these limitations in the current diagnostic paradigm suggest that research exclusively focused on refining the DSM-defined syndromes may never be successful in uncovering their underlying etiologies. For that to happen, an as yet unknown paradigm shift may need to occur."[18]

Classically, paradigm shift means a significant change in the underlying assumptions within science. For example, the acceptance that the earth rotates around the sun rather than vice versa was a famous paradigm shift in the 1600s. When the DSM-V committee said we need a paradigm shift, they were making a big statement.

While the authors of the *Research Agenda* did not define exactly what this paradigm shift would entail, they mentioned some possibilities. One idea was that a review of the latest findings in neuroscience would allow us to categorize psychiatric disease in terms of neurobiology or genetics. Another thought was to define mental disorders along a spectrum rather than as discrete categories. Instead of diagnosing someone with panic disorder or major depression, for example, perhaps a given patient could be described as scoring a 3 on anxiety, an 8 on depression, a 5 on poor concentration, and so on. Medications could then be chosen to target symptoms rather than to target static labels. In fact, this is not far from the way many psychiatrists actually make their prescribing decisions.

In 2002, when the *Research Agenda* was first published, the planned publication of DSM-V was a decade away, and there seemed to be plenty of time to nail down the specifics of the paradigm shift. But by 2008, it appeared that little had been accomplished. Robert Spitzer, the DSM pioneer who we met earlier in this chapter, became concerned and began to investigate. He wrote to both David Kupfer (the chair of DSM-V) and Darrel Regier (the vice-chair), asking them for copies of the minutes of the committee meetings.

According to Spitzer, who detailed the correspondence in one of the APA's journals,[19] they refused his request, writing him that it was "important to maintain DSM-V confidentiality." They told Spitzer that all members of DSM-V task forces were now required to sign "confidentiality agreements," preventing them from revealing the content of committee discussions unless it was "necessary for the development of DSM-V."

Outraged, Spitzer responded that "this unprecedented attempt to revise *DSM* in secrecy indicates a failure to understand that revising a diagnostic manual—as a scientific process—benefits from the very exchange of information that is prohibited by the confidentiality agreement." In the same issue, the journal published a response from Regier and the APA leadership. Saying that there was a "misunderstanding concerning the confidentiality" of the DSM process, they assured the readers that committee members were free to talk to others about the proceedings, as long as they felt it was necessary for their DSM-V work.[20]

Soon, in an apparent attempt to appease critics, the APA posted more information about the DSM-V process on its Web site, including the names of all task force members, a full disclosure of their relationships with the drug industry, and summaries of the main points being discussed.[21]

That's when all hell broke loose.

Allen Frances, another Columbia university psychiatrist, who had been the chair of the DSM-IV committee, wrote a scathing editorial for *Psychiatric Times*. Having read through the work groups' summaries and various articles about the DSM-V, Frances declared that "The work on DSM-V has, so far, displayed an unhappy combination of soaring ambition and remarkably weak methodology.[22]

"First," he wrote, "let's expose the absurdity of the DSM-V claim that it will constitute a 'paradigm shift' in psychiatric diagnosis . . ." He went on to argue that the underlying science of psychiatry has not advanced enough to merit the kind of extreme makeover proposed by the DSM-V officials:

> There can be no dramatic improvements in psychiatric diagnosis until we make a fundamental leap in our understanding of what causes mental disorders. The incredible recent advances in neuroscience, molecular biology, and brain imaging that have taught us so much about normal brain functioning are still not relevant to the clinical practicalities of everyday psychiatric diagnosis. The clearest evidence supporting this disappointing fact is that not even one biological test is ready for inclusion in the criteria sets for DSM-V.

He then systematically attacked every aspect of the paradigm shift. He said that the idea of adding symptom rating scales was poorly conceived because busy clinicians would balk at the extra paperwork. He panned most of DSM-V's proposed changes in diagnostic criteria, arguing that the evidence in support of these was slim and that the new definitions would make it too easy to diagnose patients. Two examples: a proposal for a "prepsychotic" category to identify people who might in the future develop schizophrenia, and one for "mild cognitive impairment" to identify individuals who might go on to develop Alzheimer's disease.

The result of these broadened categories, he argued, "would be a wholesale imperial medicalization of normality that will trivialize mental disorder and lead to a deluge of unneeded medication treatment—a bonanza for the pharmaceutical industry but at a huge cost to the new false positive 'patients' caught in the excessively wide DSM-V net."

Such arguments were not exactly new—Christopher Lane and others had been making them for years. But Frances's editorial was devastating because of who Allen Frances was. He was not a sociologist, or a literature professor, or a member of an antipsychiatry sect such as Scientology. He was the man who had overseen the version of DSM currently being used by millions of clinicians throughout the world. He was the establishment, and he was turning the establishment on its head.

Soon after this editorial was released, Jane Costello, a superstar in the study of child psychiatry at Duke University, announced she was resigning from her DSM-V work group. She cited essentially the same problems outlined by Frances.[23]

Suddenly, it appeared that DSM-V was imploding. In an effort to control the damage, the APA leadership published a rebuttal to Frances. Inexplicably, it concluded with a personal attack on Dr. Frances, accusing him of being motivated by greed, because a book he had coauthored on DSM-IV would not be reissued after DSM-V.[24] But Frances told the *Boston Globe* that these royalties never amounted to more than $10,000 per year.[25] It seemed, to say the least, unlikely that a world-famous psychiatrist would have written such a professionally risky editorial in order to maintain a $10,000/year sinecure.

As this book was in press, the DSM-V was still scheduled for publication sometime in 2013. It looks as though it will include no paradigm shift after all. During a phone interview, Regier told me that their initial hope of adding the neurobiological criteria to the diseases would not happen. "It's not clear that there is enough evidence," he said.[26]

But still unanswered is whether certain diagnoses will be substantially broadened, and whether Dr. Frances's concern that it will be a bonanza for the pharmaceutical industry is true. There's no question that fortunes can be made based on seemingly minor additions. For example, the DSM-V work group on neurocognitive disorders is considering adding a new diagnosis called "mild cognitive impairment" (MCI), which is a kind of pre-dementia category. These are patients who complain of poor memory that is not severe enough to qualify for the diagnosis of dementia. But they are at high risk: about 10 percent of patients with MCI develop dementia per year.[27]

If MCI became a full-fledged DSM diagnosis, the results could be positive or negative, and probably a little of both. On the one hand, patients with significant memory problems could be given a diagnostic label and a better sense of their prognosis. For some patients and family members, even this little bit of knowledge is reassuring. On the other hand, there is the danger of over-diagnosis. A certain degree of memory loss is normal with aging, and most older people with absentmindedness have a benign condition termed "age-associated memory impairment," and are at no higher risk for dementia.[28] Once MCI gains a foothold in DSM-V, doctors are likely to look more zealously for the disorder and may generate false positive diagnoses. And once patients receive this diagnosis, they are likely to receive a trial of an anti-dementia drug (such as

Aricept) even though such drugs have not been shown to prevent dementia in MCI patients.[29] Pharmaceutical companies, when motivated by the scent of a vast new market, have proven themselves adept at trumping up meager findings in order to convince doctors to prescribe their drugs.

The DSM and pharmaceutical companies have long been engaged in a symbiotic dance, with each partner supporting the other. The proliferation of diagnostic labels has proved crucial for the growth of the pharmaceutical industry. When a new diagnosis is published, drug companies flock to treat potential new customers, in a psychopharmacologic land grab. In turn, the DSM brand is strengthened, because drug companies will promote the new condition in their advertising (they will often call this "medical education"), having the effect of encouraging clinicians to purchase the latest version of the manual.

The profusion of diagnoses has unquestionably yielded benefits, encouraging companies to develop new drugs for real conditions. Before DSM-III, for example, if a drug company wanted to test a new compound for anxiety, it would enroll patients diagnosed with "anxiety neurosis," which would yield a hodgepodge of patients with differing symptoms, such as panic disorder, generalized anxiety disorder, and PTSD. If a drug worked for the entire group, it was not clear which condition it targeted the best. DSM-III provided the criteria researchers could use to enroll only patients with, say, panic disorder into a drug trial. This advance, in turn, meant that companies could speed up the process of winning FDA approval of drugs for psychiatric disorders.

Overall, I believe that the development of these new drugs was a good thing, because the treatments available at the time (mainly psychoanalytic therapy) could do little to treat these symptoms. Through the 1980s and 1990s, drugs were developed that were effective for a range of problems, including depression, anxiety disorders, and schizophrenia. But gradually, the pharmaceutical industry became turbocharged, and began feeding off of the new diagnostic labels being defined by DSM committee members.

The best example of this is the progression of "me-too" drugs, especially in the category of the Prozac-like drugs, designated SSRIs. After Prozac's success, other companies created their own compounds that were minor molecular variations. Working off of the new DSM diagnoses, they paid for clinical studies showing that their SSRI was effective not only for depression, like Prozac, but also for some other disorders. GlaxoSmithKline, for example, conducted studies showing that its SSRI, Paxil, was effective for depression, panic disorder, obsessive compulsive disorder, generalized anxiety disorder, post-traumatic stress disorder, and social anxiety disorder.[30] Each new indication was accompanied by expensive advertising campaigns touting yet another reason to prescribe Paxil rather than one of its competitors. In reality, all psychiatrists have come to realize that all the SSRIs—there are now about ten on the market, depending on how you categorize a particular drug—work pretty much equivalently, regardless of which formal "indications" the FDA has approved.

In the next two chapters, I will explore how psychiatrists think about the drugs we prescribe, and how our conceptions and our practices have been manipulated by drug company marketing strategies. Unfortunately, we know a good bit less about what we are doing than you might think.

Chapter 4

How Medications Became the New Therapy

As the psychopharmacologist and historian David Healy has written, "Specific diseases are of no use without specific cures."[1] The cures have come to us in the form of an avalanche of medications from pharmaceutical companies, and in response, since the mid-1990s, psychiatrists have gone on a binge of drug prescribing unprecedented in history.

In 1996, 13 million Americans were taking an antidepressant; nine years later, in 2005, that number had more than doubled, to 27 million. One in ten Americans over the age of six is now taking an antidepressant.[2] Other mind medications are on the rise as well. The use of sleeping pills doubled from 2000 to 2004, and in 2006 it was estimated that 8.6 million Americans used the medications regularly.[3] Stimulants like Ritalin and Dexedrine are also a growth industry, with 5 percent of American children taking stimulants every day.[4]

When stated in such bald terms, these figures sound like a call to arms, but why should they? Prescriptions of new medications for diabetes, coronary artery disease, and infectious diseases have also soared over the last few decades. Most view this as a sign of medical progress. Why do the figures on psychiatric drugs strike us more negatively? Are we overdoing psychiatric treatment, or are we simply entering a brave new world of psychiatry, in which we have developed pills to treat every conceivable complaint? The answers to these questions are complex.

To try to get to the truth, let's start with a typical success story of modern psychopharmacology. James, a man in his late thirties, was referred to me by his family practitioner. He told me he was feeling trapped in his teaching job, dissatisfied with his marriage, and generally unhappy with every aspect of his life. Every morning, he woke up at 4 a.m., dreading what the day would bring. He'd been assigned a student teacher who believed she was God's gift to pedagogy, and she had suggested four separate projects for his fifth-grade classroom, any one of which would create a good deal more work for him. He was exhausted, dragging through his days, barely concealing his frustration with everyone around him.

"Every day is another nightmare," he told me during that first visit.

When he returned home, he wanted to flop down on the couch and watch TV in order to quell the worry that began building up throughout the night as he contemplated his next day. His wife usually got home from work later, and she had taken to giving him icy looks when she saw him planted in front of the tube, not doing anything about dinner.

I diagnosed James with major depression as well as anxiety. He needed both medication and therapy. When he left his first session, he was carrying three prescriptions I had written for him: Celexa for depression, Ativan for anxiety, and Ambien for insomnia. A month later, at his next appointment, he was already feeling somewhat better. He was gaining perspective on things. He was viewing his wife less as an opponent and more as a partner. But he had a couple of new problems. First, beginning in the early afternoon, he was dog-tired, ready to take a nap at a moment's notice. Second, he had less sex drive, and when he did have sex, he felt like, as he put it, "I'm wearing a sock down there." Orgasms felt about as exciting as brushing his teeth.

Both fatigue and lowered libido are common side effects of Celexa and other SSRIs. But since the medication appeared to be helping his depression, I was reluctant to discontinue it. So I decided to treat the side effects with other medications—chasing the tail, as it were. For his fatigue, I prescribed Provigil, a wakefulness-enhancing drug, and for his erectile dysfunction, I prescribed that great sponsor of *Monday Night Football*, Viagra. James was now on five medications, and this cocktail seemed to do the trick. Over the next few months, his mood came back to normal, he had more energy since taking Provigil (though sometimes it caused him to be too hyper), he found the Viagra helpful (it gave him headaches, but he could take Tylenol for that), he used the Ativan occasionally for anxiety, and he often popped an Ambien to put him to sleep. As far as therapy, James said he hadn't contacted anyone. "The meds are working fine," he reported in visit after visit.

James, five medications and all, is the type of patient who makes psychiatrists love to prescribe drugs. For him, everything clicked. I could sit back and admire the results, as one might admire a fine work of art.

But there is also something about James that seems unsettling. Yes, his medication regimen is helping him to feel happier and to move on with his life. But the way his emotions are cobbled together by medications, with drugs to treat the side effects of the original drugs, gives him a fragile appearance. It reminds me of the pickup trucks I sometimes see on the back roads of New Hampshire, just north of my town. New Englanders, famous for their thrift and ingenuity, have found ways to keep these old Fords and Chevys on the road forever. Cabs might be tied on to chassis with baling wire; torn seats are mended with duct tape; engines are rebuilt one cylinder at a time. When you see these jalopies driving around, you marvel that they are still on the road, but you wonder what would happen if one crucial piece of wiring were to snap one day. Would the vehicle simply fall apart into a pile of rubber and metal and glass?

For James, the duct tape meds, those I used to treat side effects, worked well. But sometimes they create problems of their own. For example, James's Ambien was first approved by the FDA in 1992 and was billed as the first of an entirely new class of sleeping pills, which would cause no sensation of being high and therefore no addiction. But it has not turned out that way. Not only has Ambien become a popular drug of abuse, it leads to bizarre side effects such as sleep-walking, sleep-driving, and sleep-eating, side effects rarely seen with older sleeping pills like Valium.[5]

Recently, for example, one of my patients, a young working woman with no children, came in for a regular medication visit. One of her medications was Ambien, and I asked her if it had been helpful for her insomnia. "I'm not sure it's the right medication for me, doctor," she began. "I think it's doing some strange things."

"Please explain."

"I took it the other night and went to sleep fine, then I woke up and went to work. At work, I got a call from an ex-boyfriend, someone I hadn't seen in a couple of years. He asked me if I was 'okay.' I asked why he was asking. He said I had called him at four in the morning, crying, telling him that I loved him. I have no memory at all of doing that."

Other patients have told me that they wake up in the morning to kitchen counters strewn with sandwich fixings, with no memory of having gorged in the middle of the night. This led one woman to develop a significant weight gain problem before I stopped the Ambien.

Many of my patients seem tentatively held together by a patchwork of new medications whose mechanisms of action are mysterious and whose side effects are still being discovered. We target discrete symptoms with treatments, and other drugs are piled on top to treat side effects. I wonder whether the essence of the psychological problem is really being addressed; generally, modern psychiatry has no way of even understanding what the "underlying problem" might be. In treating emotional problems with medications, I worry that we are discouraging patients from learning life skills that they could use to truly solve their problems.

If James represents a psychopharmacological success story, Nancy represents a more typical case, and exemplifies the limitations of our knowledge and the haphazard way psychiatrists often make decisions about treatment. Nancy is a married woman in her fifties who worked as a receptionist at an insurance company and who was referred to me for a medication evaluation by her therapist. She told me that she had struggled with depression and anxiety off and on for years. She had been raised in a large family by a mother who had once been admitted to a psychiatric hospital for what was then called a nervous breakdown (in modern terminology, this might have been an episode of depression or bipolar disorder) and a father who drank a fair amount, but who maintained a steady job and was never violent toward his family. Nancy married young, and had one daughter and several grandchildren. Her husband was a polite but emotionally distant man who had recently retired, while Nancy maintained her part-time job.

She had first sought therapy a couple of years earlier because she and her daughter were arguing about how much time and energy Nancy wanted to devote to handling her daughter's child care needs. While Nancy loved her energetic young grandson, he was a challenge to supervise, and she felt exploited and underappreciated by her daughter, who appeared to take her mother's assistance for granted. She was also anxious about her job, though apparently irrationally so. Her boss called her a model employee, but Nancy second-guessed herself and felt overwhelmed by her responsibilities.

Despite weekly psychotherapy, Nancy's anxiety had mounted. Occasionally, she would have panic attacks, but more often she felt a queasy kind of stomach tension. She was irritable and unhappy. I ran through the DSM-IV criteria of depression, and she had insomnia, poor concentration, a lack of pleasure, and poor energy and motivation. She had never thought about suicide, but she often wished she could just "go away and disappear."

She had already gone to her primary care doctor, who had ordered blood tests and a cardiogram, all of which were normal. Assuring her that this was not a medical problem, I diagnosed her with major depression and generalized anxiety disorder, and we discussed medications. In a patient with depression and anxiety, there are at least twenty drugs to choose from, and all of them are equivalently effective. About a dozen of these are considered "second-generation" antidepressants, because they were introduced more recently and have fewer side effects than the original tricyclics and MAOIs. These newer medications include Prozac, Paxil, Paxil CR, Zoloft, Celexa, Lexapro, Luvox, Luvox CR, Effexor XR, Cymbalta, Wellbutrin, Remeron, and Serzone. How is one to decide?

A therapist friend of mine, Susan Hochstedler, who often refers patients for medication treatment, has heard her clients talk about psychiatrists as though they are sophisticated auto mechanics: "Patients think their psychiatrist can open up their brain like the hood of a car and check various dipsticks," she said. " 'Yep, it looks like your serotonin is low, we'll need to top that off with a little Prozac, but your dopamine is fine, we'll check that again in six months.'"

Of course, this is not the way it works. While it is true that most of our drugs affect neurotransmitters in various ways, when psychiatrists start using what I call neurobabble, beware, because we rarely know what we are talking about. I fall into this habit with patients all the time. When I find myself using phrases like "chemical imbalance" and "serotonin deficiency," it is usually because I'm trying to convince a reluctant patient to take a medication. Using these words makes their illness seem more biological, taking some of the stigma away from having a mental illness. The implicit message I deliver in using such language is "Your illness is biological, it is not your fault, and you are not going to be able to cure it by thinking it away."

Indeed, how could mental illness not be, ultimately, biological? All thoughts and emotions come from the brain, and so disordered thoughts and emotions must come from a disordered brain. But few laypeople realize how little we actually know about the underpinnings of these disorders.

In order to appreciate the extent of our ignorance, you need to know some basics of neuroscience.[6] The human brain is famously made up of 100 billion nerve cells, or neurons. Neurons communicate with one another by squirting chemicals into the gaps separating them from other neurons, called synapses. These chemicals are termed "neurotransmitters," and each one travels quickly to another neuron, where it locates its molecular mirror image embedded in the receiving neuron's skin, or membrane. The mirror image molecule is called a "receptor," and each neuron is studded with thousands of such receptors. Like keys fitting precisely into locks, a given neurotransmitter, such as serotonin, fits into a serotonin receptor. Norepinephrine fits into a norepinephrine receptor, dopamine fits into a dopamine receptor, and so on.

Once this landing has occurred, the receiving neuron undergoes a dramatic change. Immediately, its entire membrane becomes porous, allowing atoms in the surrounding fluid to rush into the neuron's interior. These inrushing particles are all electrically charged, and this sudden change in the neuron's voltage causes it to "fire." When a neuron fires, it releases its own supply of neurotransmitters into surrounding synapses. These neurotransmitters, in turn, find other neurons to land on, causing these neurons to fire. Like a chemical and electrical game of dominos, firing neurons propagate a rapid succession of other firing neurons. These cascades are, essentially, what cause us to have our thoughts, perceptions, and emotions. This much we feel confident we've worked out.

We also know that because neurotransmitters are so crucial to how our brains function, our neurons have developed elaborate mechanisms to maintain a good supply of them. We are constantly creating new neurotransmitters from raw molecular materials. In addition, our brains have a system for recycling the neurotransmitters that we have just released—"transporter pumps" that vacuum up used chemicals for storage and eventual reuse.

And this is where the common antidepressants come into play. All of the SSRI antidepressants—Prozac, Paxil, Zoloft, Luvox, Celexa, and Lexapro—temporarily disable the serotonin transporter pumps, thereby allowing serotonin to stay in the neural gap longer, resulting in higher levels. This is why they are called "specific serotonin reuptake inhibitors"—because they specifically disable the serotonin pump, rather than the pumps for other neurotransmitters.

Other antidepressants are variations on this theme. For example, Effexor and Cymbalta are termed "SNRIs," or serotonin norepinephrine reuptake inhibitors, disabling the vacuum cleaners for both serotonin and norepinephrine. For this reason, they are sometimes also called "dual reuptake inhibitors."

The idea that depression is a "chemical imbalance" derives from how the drugs seem to work. We have come to the theory through a process of deduction, reasoning backward from the effects antidepressants have on neurotransmitters. Antidepressants increase levels of neurotransmitters in the synapses, and they treat depression. Ergo, depression must be caused by a *deficiency* of such neurotransmitters. Officially, this theory of depression is called the "monoamine hypothesis," because the deficient neurotransmitters, serotonin and norepinephrine, are chemically classified as monoamines.

The theory makes intuitive sense, explaining its enduring popularity. But the problem is that there is no *direct* evidence that a serotonin or norepinephrine deficiency is involved, despite thousands of studies that have attempted to demonstrate such a deficiency.[7] Notice that I do not say that there is *no* evidence for the monoamine hypothesis. Over the years, tantalizing findings have surfaced here and there. But the problem is that getting precise measures of brain neurotransmitters has proven devilishly tricky.

You can't just put a syringe into a living brain and draw out fluid without damaging brain tissue, and even if you could, levels of serotonin in a brain humming with neural activity are likely to ebb and flow unpredictably. Thus, scientists have had to settle for indirect measurements, such as the breakdown products in the blood, urine, or cerebrospinal fluid (CSF). Another indirect, if more gruesome, method entails removing brains from bodies after death, grinding up the neurons, and measuring levels of neurotransmitters postmortem. Though some results have been suggestive, all these studies thus far have been inconclusive. The most recent definitive review of all basic antidepressant research, published in the *New England Journal of Medicine*, stated this clearly: "Numerous studies of norepinephrine and serotonin metabolites in plasma, urine, and cerebrospinal fluid, as well as postmortem studies of the brains of patients with depression, have yet to identify the purported deficiency reliably."[8]

Stymied by one avenue of research, scientists have been creative. For example, researchers have created special drinks that deplete levels of serotonin or norepinephrine when imbibed.[9] Theoretically, if depression were caused by a depletion of these chemicals, these potions should lead to deep and certain gloom. But it has not panned out that way. When normal people drink these potions, their moods do not change at all. Similarly, the drinks don't cause depressed patients to become any more depressed than they are already. However, when *recovered* depressed patients drink the potions, they sometimes suffer what the researchers call "transient depressive symptoms," though not full-blown major depression. The results of these depletion studies imply strongly that low neurotransmitters are unlikely to be the cause of depression; nonetheless, alterations in these chemicals probably have some genuine role in treatment, at least for some patients.

Another challenge to the chemical imbalance theory is the well-known delay in the effect of antidepressants—in most patients, these drugs take at least two weeks before they begin to work. Yet, the drugs begin altering levels of serotonin and norepinephrine immediately. In order to explain this, authorities have created increasingly elaborate theories about "downstream" effects of antidepressants, in which neurotransmitters set into motion a cascade of biochemical events that eventually cause genes to be activated. Again, the theories are ingenious but unproven.

There are similarly elaborate chemical imbalance theories of the other major mental illnesses. For years, the going explanation for schizophrenia was the "dopamine hypothesis."[10] Because antipsychotics block the action of the neurotransmitter dopamine, it seemed reasonable to presume that psychosis must be caused by too much dopamine. You can't measure dopamine directly in the brain, but you can measure the main by-product in the spinal fluid. More than a dozen studies have compared levels of dopamine metabolites in schizophrenics versus normal controls; in most studies, there were no differences, and in a few, the levels were *lower* in schizophrenics, exactly the *opposite* of what would be predicted by the dopamine hypothesis.[11] Other studies, looking at postmortem brains or PET scans of living patients, have been inconclusive, partly because most of the patients studied have already been taking antipsychotics. This means that any alterations found in dopamine receptors are as likely to be an artifact of the medication as they are to reflect the underlying cause of schizophrenia.

"As it turns out, there is very little evidence that the dopamine system is truly abnormal in schizophrenia, or if it is abnormal, this may well be the consequence of completely different brain pathology," according to Dr. Dost Ongur, who directs the Schizophrenia and Bipolar Disorder Program at McLean Hospital.[12] Ongur believes that while blocking dopamine might indeed help to quiet hallucinations, the implications for the neurobiology are unclear.

"As an analogy," he explained, "imagine being in a room that is too hot because there is a big fire in the fireplace. If you can't see the fireplace, you would not know that this is the source of the heat, and you might open a window to cool it down. The room cools down a bit, and you might say, 'The cause of the heat in the room is the windows,' but in fact the actual cause is the fire, and opening the window is only palliative. Similarly, blocking dopamine receptors helps alleviate schizophrenia but the root cause of the psychotic symptoms may have little to do with dopamine."

There is no shortage of alternative theories. Writing in the journal *Schizophrenia Research*, four luminaries in the field reviewed dozens of recent findings in an article aptly titled "Schizophrenia, 'just the facts': What we know in 2008." Stuggling to synthesize the hodgepodge of theories, they compared present-day researchers to the proverbial blind men, each of whom touched a different part of an elephant in order to identify the mysterious object. Each came up with different conclusions, but all missed the big picture—that this was an elephant. To make matters even more complex, they said, there may well be different versions of schizophrenia: "All these theorists might be assuming that there is one elephant that everyone could see, if only they were unblinded. However, we argue that even this assumption could well be wrong, and that there might be more than one elephant, or some other animals we do not know of."[13]

The neuroscientists are well-intentioned, and are pushing our basic understanding of mental illness gradually forward. But it is crucial that we realize how much we know and how much we do not know. In virtually all of the psychiatric disorders—including depression, schizophrenia, bipolar disorder, and anxiety disorders—the shadow of our ignorance overwhelms the few dim lights of our knowledge.

What about the genetics of mental illness? Genetics is hot lately. The Human Genome Project deciphered our genes nearly a decade ago, and private companies have adapted these findings for home genetic test kits to tell us our risk of developing heart disease, cancer, and diabetes.[14]

Here, too, we have been stymied by the complexity of the brain. For example, in 2003, researchers caused a flurry of excitement by announcing the results of a genetic study of 847 patients with depression. It appeared that patients who had a gene variant that interfered with serotonin transport had up to triple the normal risk of becoming depressed after stressful life events, such as a divorce or a lost job.[15] If replicated, this result would have allowed us to identify patients who are particularly prone to depression, potentially allowing us to prevent the disorder. Six years later, however, a different group of researchers reviewed data from 14 other genetic studies of more than 14,000 depressed patients, to see how the 2003 finding held up. They were careful to review all the papers ever published on this topic (including the original paper) and they combined the data in a statistical procedure called a meta-analysis. They concluded that: "This meta-analysis yielded no evidence that the serotonin transporter genotype alone or in interaction with stressful life events is associated with an elevated risk of depression in men alone, women alone, or in both sexes combined."[16]

Thud. Talk about a scientific buzz kill. Kenneth Kendler, one of the leading researchers in psychiatric genetics, expressed the disappointment of much of the profession: "This is another example of getting a bit of wind knocked out of our sails. The bottom line here has been that finding genes that impact on human behavior has proven to be very difficult. The field has on many occasions been overly optimistic."[17]

There is no question that psychiatric problems can be inherited—we know this from studies comparing identical twins with fraternal twins. Identical twins are genetically the same, meaning that they share 100 percent of their DNA, whereas nonidentical (fraternal) twins share only 50 percent of their genes. Studies looking at the concordance rate of schizophrenia—that is, how commonly *both* siblings develop the same disorder—have found a concordance rate of 10 percent in nonidentical twins, versus 40 percent in identical twins.[18] This implies that genetics plays a significant role in schizophrenia. But what is that role? Answering this question has been devilishly hard, and the latest landmark study found that we are much further away from identifying such genes than we ever thought.

In this study (actually, a series of three studies reported at the same time), researchers compared the genetic sequences of 10,000 patients with schizophrenia to 20,000 normal people.[19] This technique, called "genome-wide scans," would not have been possible several years ago, before superpowered computer-based genetic research techniques were developed. The results? On the plus side they did in fact identify the specific genes residing in schizophrenia DNA. Unfortunately, they found an embarrassment of riches—over 10,000 gene variants appear to have a role in "causing" schizophrenia. The bottom line, according to *New York Times* science blogger Nicholas Wade, is that "Schizophrenia . . . seems to be not a single disease, but the end point of 10,000 different disruptions to the delicate architecture of the human brain. Yes, that discovery is a landmark. The kind that says you have 10,000 miles yet to go."[20]

Undoubtedly, there are both neurobiological and genetic causes for all mental disorders, but they are still beyond our understanding. Rather than telling patients that depression is caused by a chemical imbalance, we could more accurately say, "Depression, and all mental illness, must be caused by something that has gone wrong in the brain. We have some promising ideas, but we don't have an answer yet. Luckily, we've stumbled upon several drugs that seem to help a great deal."

Obviously, this rendition doesn't inspire a great deal of confidence in your doctor or in the medication being prescribed. For this reason, in order to build up more consumer confidence in their drugs, companies still use the neurotransmitter deficiency hypothesis in direct-to-consumer ads. Thus, for example, Forest Pharmaceuticals, the maker of Lexapro, says: "Lexapro appears to work by increasing the available supply of serotonin." Eli Lilly has this to say about Cymbalta: "Although the way Cymbalta works in people is not fully known, medical experts believe it increases the activity of two naturally occurring substances in the brain called serotonin and norepinephrine."[21]

Who can blame these companies? Both psychiatrists and our patients want to believe that we have a basic understanding of what we are doing. Drug companies are happy to oblige, because offering a mechanism of action can become a valuable part of the medication's branding strategy. Effexor, for example, has long advertised itself as being a dual reuptake inhibitor, thereby bolstering its claims that it is more effective than SSRIs. After all, doesn't it make sense that increasing levels of two neurotransmitters is better than one?

The problem is that we have no evidence that simply piling on neurotransmitters yields any benefit.

Choosing the right medication for a given patient is crucial, but thus far we are lacking the knowledge to make such choices scientifically. Instead, we rely on the "art" of prescribing—a series of rules of thumb with some backup from clinical studies here and there. Returning to Nancy, I ended up choosing the SSRI Zoloft for her. Why? I'm not entirely sure, though I could drum up some reasons. I could say that Zoloft has a good side-effect profile, that it doesn't interact with other drugs, and that it has a long track record. But I could make the same arguments for Celexa or Lexapro. A colleague across town might have chosen Effexor, or Wellbutrin, or Serzone, and could have provided a good rationale for any of those choices as well. To a remarkable degree, our choice of medications is subjective, even random. Perhaps your psychiatrist is in a Lexapro mood this morning, because he was just visited by an attractive Lexapro drug rep. Or maybe he is in a Prozac mood, because a relative of his took it recently and did well. In truth, it didn't really matter which antidepressant I chose for Nancy, because they are equally likely to target her symptoms.

The essentially random nature of drug prescribing is attested to by the American Psychiatric Association's treatment guidelines for depression. If you were a psychiatrist seeking advice from the APA for what to prescribe for a patient like Nancy, here is what you would read: "The following medications are likely to be optimal agents for most patients: SSRIs, desipramine, nortriptyline, bupropion, and venlafaxine."[22] In other words, pick a drug, any drug.

The fact is that psychopharmacology is primarily trial and error, a kind of muddling through different candidate medications until we hit on one that works. We prescribe medications to treat symptoms that our patients tell us about, and we rely largely on intangible factors to make these decisions.

A month or so after I had prescribed Nancy her medication, she came into my office with a smile. "I'm a nicer person on Zoloft," she said. She was less irritable, and more in control of her emotions. Life began to settle down.

But eventually her symptoms resurfaced. "I crashed over the holidays," she said during a January appointment. Family tensions had flared up over an unpleasant Christmas dinner, and she had stormed away from the table in order to calm down. Over the next several weeks, she replayed the scene in her mind again and again. Despite her Zoloft and weekly psychotherapy, she was unable to shake a sense of discouragement and free-floating anxiety. We were faced with another medication decision. What to do in a case like this, in which the first drug loses its effectiveness?

The process of selecting a second agent is guesswork. A few years ago, in order to help doctors decide what to do next in situations like Nancy's (which is common in psychiatric practice), NIMH (the National Institute of Mental Health) funded a $35 million study that enrolled over four thousand patients with depression. It was the largest psychiatric clinical trial in history. All four thousand patients were started on the SSRI Celexa. After eight weeks, about half of them improved. The next phase of the study was the crucial part, though. Those patients who did *not* improve on Celexa were assigned to one of two different options. In the first option (called the "switch option"), Celexa was discontinued, and the patients were given one of three popular antidepressants—Wellbutrin SR, Effexor XR, or Zoloft. In the second option (called "augmentation"), patients stayed on the ineffective Celexa, and a second medication was added (either Wellbutrin SR or BuSpar).

For psychiatrists practicing in the trenches, this was a beautifully designed study, because, unlike most drug trials that simply put newly depressed patients on a single drug and compare it with placebo, this study would help us decide what to do when the first drug did not work. Because this is a situation that comes up so often, the results were anticipated with an excitement that I had rarely seen in the field.

But unfortunately, the results were disappointing—there were no differences between *any* of the second-step strategies used. Whether patients were switched to Wellbutrin, Effexor, or Zoloft didn't matter—all three treatments yielded the same 25 percent remission rate. When patients were assigned to the add-on strategy, there was no clear difference between Wellbutrin and BuSpar.[23]

These results were a double blow to psychiatrists. First, they provided us with no rationale for choosing one medication strategy over another. Second, and more fundamentally, the results implied that we don't have a handle on the mechanisms of action of antidepressants. A common practice in medicating patients is to start with an SSRI, and if that doesn't work, to choose a drug with a different mechanism of action. But this study did not support this practice. Drugs with completely different effects on neurotransmitters worked equivalently—and in this case, not particularly well.

Antidepressants do differ in one important way, though—side effects. Thus, for example, SSRIs usually cause patients some amount of sexual dysfunction, such as impotence in men or anorgasmia in women, whereas Wellbutrin almost never causes this problem. Wellbutrin, however, has its own liability, which is that in high doses it can cause seizures. Other antidepressants, such as Paxil or Remeron, are also great sleeping pills, but at the cost of possible weight gain. This makes them perfect medications for patients who have insomnia and are underweight, but not good choices for many other people.

In Nancy's case, I did the simplest thing possible—I increased her dose of Zoloft from the original 50 mg/day to 100 mg/day. When that didn't work, I went up to 150 mg/day. The rationale here is obvious—if 50 mg is good, 100 mg is better. Scientifically, there are few studies to prove this intuitively appealing rule of thumb. Drug manufacturers often compare different initial dosages of their antidepressants and the results are generally that higher and lower doses work about the same, though there is some variation. But the studies to truly answer the question of whether escalating a dose is better have rarely been done. In such studies, you would have to follow a large group of patients who have started on a given dose (like Nancy's 50 mg of Zoloft), who have lost their response and then are randomly assigned to either continuing the same dose or to a higher dose. Then you would test them a month later to see if the one strategy worked any better than the other. Few such studies have been done, and the results have varied, so we are left to our own devices and hunches in these situations.

After Nancy's Zoloft was increased, her mood brightened temporarily, but a few months later, she worsened, and I decided to switch her to Celexa and to add Ativan, a tranquilizer. Her anxiety eased, but the Celexa caused her to feel slowed down and apathetic ("I feel like a zombie," she said). I tried Effexor. The Celexa-induced zombie feeling went away, but her mood stayed somewhat low. I proposed other medication options, but Nancy wanted to take a break from this parade of drugs, and I could hardly blame her. "I can live with how I'm feeling," she said. "I'm tired of being a guinea pig." We decided to stick with Effexor and Ativan.

Such is modern psychopharmacology. Guided purely by symptoms, we try different drugs, with no real conception of what we are trying to fix, or of how the drugs are working. I am perpetually astonished that we are so effective for so many patients. The way we prescribe medication reminds me of the "Fonzarelli Fix" in the sitcom *Happy Days*. When confronted with a broken jukebox or TV, Arthur "The Fonz" Fonzarelli, the cool heartthrob dressed in T-shirt and black leather jacket, would simply give it a good bash on the side, and the machine would inevitably spring back to life.

That our versions of the Fonzarelli Fix work so well is a tribute to that magical force in the history of medicine, serendipity. All major categories of psychiatric drugs were originally discovered by accident.

Drugs by Accident

The first antipsychotic, Thorazine, was discovered not by a psychiatrist but by an army surgeon named Henri Laborit.[24] Laborit happened upon Thorazine in his quest for a better antihistamine. At the time, in the 1940s, one of the main causes of death on the operating table was surgical shock, which refers to a rapid and lethal loss of blood pressure. Shock was sometimes a side effect of the anesthesia drugs used at the time, and one theory about the cause was that excessive amounts of histamine were released into the bloodstream.

Laborit and others experimented with giving patients antihistamines before surgery and found that, indeed, they seemed to lower the frequency of shock. In search of even more effective antihistamines, Laborit contacted a major French pharmaceutical company, Rhone-Poulenc. The company sent him an experimental compound dubbed RP4560 (the "RP" stood for Rhone-Poulenc), and Laborit tried it for his surgical patients. He found it effective, and he was also struck by an unexpected psychological side effect. While antihistamines commonly caused sleepiness, patients on RP4560 were more than drowsy; they became, to use Laborit's term, "indifferent."

Intrigued, Laborit thought this side effect could be exploited as a tranquilizer, and he urged psychiatrists at his army hospital to try it on their patients with manic depression and schizophrenia. It turned out that RP4560 was remarkably effective for treating the hallucinations and delusions of patients with schizophrenia.

Schizophrenia is a harrowing condition that remains a medical mystery, but the suffering of patients with the disorder is clear as crystal—or perhaps the better analogy would be jagged glass. I have a patient, John, who has suffered this illness since he was a teenager. He comes to my office once a month, and he smiles briefly when I greet him, sits down, and begins glancing furtively around my office, all the while mumbling something to himself.

"So how have you been, John?" I ask, but often he seems oblivious to the fact that I am addressing him. "John?"

"Oh—yes, Dr. Carlat?"

"What's going on in your head right now?"

"Oh, I don't know, Dr. Carlat."

"Were you hearing voices?"

"Yes, I hear voices."

"What are they saying to you?"

"All kinds of things. Bad things. 'You're a bad person. You can't do anything. You don't know what you're doing.'"

"Do they make you feel bad?" But he doesn't respond, because he is already swallowed back up into this world of hallucinations.

John lives in a state-subsidized apartment and has been on a dizzying array of medications. He is now on Clozaril, which is considered the most effective medication for schizophrenia, and while he is still actively symptomatic, he has been able to stay out of the hospital for the past few years.

The disease varies dramatically in outcome. One of my other patients with schizophrenia, a woman who is also on Clozaril, maintains a full-time job and is going to graduate school. Most people would not detect anything abnormal about her on a first meeting. But when she misses her medication she becomes paranoid, believing that other drivers on the road are exchanging hidden communications with their headlights and turn signals—all of it part of a conspiracy to have her killed.

All of the antipsychotic medications for this condition have evolved from the antihistamine first used by Laborit, which was eventually marketed in the United States under the brand name "Thorazine" (the generic name is chlorpromazine). Over the ensuing decades, companies have tinkered with the structure of Thorazine to produce other antipsychotics, such as Haldol, and, more recently, so-called "atypical antipsychotics" like Risperdal, Zyprexa, and Abilify.

Once it became clear that antihistamines could treat schizophrenia, psychiatrists wondered if drugs acting the same way could treat other conditions, such as depression. While Thorazine proved not to be helpful for this condition, another company, Geigy, tweaked the structure of Thorazine slightly and came up with "G22355," which would eventually be called imipramine. Thorazine and imipramine are so similar that if you put their chemical structures side by side, you can barely notice a difference. Nonetheless, when the Swiss psychiatrist Roland Kuhn tried it on forty depressed patients, the response, according to Kuhn, was "absolutely incredible, so exciting." Patients who had been confined to their hospital beds with a gloomy lethargy and no hope of cure were suddenly able to "amuse themselves and take part in the general life of the hospital, to write letters and interest themselves again in their family circumstances."

Imipramine was introduced to the market in 1958 with the brand name Tofranil, and other companies quickly came up with their own me-too versions of the drug, including amitriptyline, desipramine, and nortriptyline. Eventually, neuroscientists worked out that these drugs blocked the reuptake of serotonin and norepinephrine, and using this knowledge, Eli Lilly scientists decided to make a drug that affected primarily serotonin. And thus, in 1988, Prozac and the family of SSRIs were born.

But the most amazing example of accidental discovery involved lithium, the first drug used for bipolar disorder. Bipolar disorder is a difficult condition for laypeople to understand, because it is defined by moods that sound positive—periods of extreme happiness and high energy that are technically termed "manic episodes." However, these episodes are several steps beyond common happiness. One of the most eloquent descriptions of mania in literature is from the psychologist Kay Jamison, who described her manic episodes in her memoir, *An Unquiet Mind*:

> When you're high it's tremendous. The ideas and feelings are fast and frequent like shooting stars, and you follow them until you find better and brighter ones. Shyness goes, the right words and gestures are suddenly there, the power to captivate others a felt certainty. There are interests found in uninteresting people. Sensuality is pervasive and the desire to seduce and be seduced irresistible. Feelings of ease, intensity, power, well-being, financial omnipotence, and euphoria pervade one's marrow. But, somewhere, this changes. The fast ideas are far too fast, and there are far too many; overwhelming confusion replaces clarity. Memory goes. Humor and absorption on friends' faces are replaced by fear and concern. Everything previously moving with the grain is now against—you are irritable, angry, frightened, uncontrollable, and enmeshed totally in the blackest caves of the mind. You never knew those caves were there. It will never end, for madness carves its own reality.[25]

Jamison captures both the appeal and dangers of mania. The mind accelerates with joy, but this can last only so long. Typically, after a bout of frenetic activity, patients will crash into a depression so deep and so chronic that suicide beckons as a viable option. The lifetime rate of suicide attempts is 70 percent in patients with bipolar disorder, higher than any other mental illness.

The first treatment for this condition was discovered in 1949 by John Cade, a thirty-seven-year-old psychiatrist working at a hospital in the Australian outback. Cade was fascinated by bipolar disorder, but there was little he could do to help his patients other than to restrain them and to give them tranquilizers. The manic episodes reminded him of hyperthyroidism, in which patients developed anxiety, excessive energy, and other maniclike symptoms due to an overproduction of thyroid hormone. He reasoned that the mania of bipolar disorder might, like hyperthyroidism, be triggered by the overproduction of some biological "substance."

Working alone in an unused hospital kitchen, Cade began a series of experiments in which he injected the urine of manic patients into guinea pigs to see if it would cause them to exhibit a guinea pig equivalent of mania. However, many of the animals died, and Cade speculated that the uric acid in the urine, which crystallized, might be the culprit. So he ordered a well-known solvent, lithium, to help keep the uric acid safely dissolved.

Cade mixed the lithium into the urine of the bipolar patients, and then injected this into the guinea pigs. The animals survived, but far from becoming manic, they became sedated. On a whim, Cade injected them with lithium alone, and again, the animals were apathetic and sedated, suggesting that it was the lithium, and not the bipolar patients' urine, that had possessed the pharmacologic quality. He decided to try lithium on his manic patients, and he published a detailed description of their response in the *Medical Journal of Australia* in 1949.[26]

In the understated tone typical of journal articles, Cade wrote that the response of his patients "was gratifying." In reading through the cases, the more appropriate term would be "miraculous." Case I, for example, identified as "W.B.," was a fifty-one-year-old man who had been manic continuously for five years. He had been living on the hospital ward all that time, and Cade wrote that he had been in a "state of chronic manic excitement," was "restless, dirty, destructive," and had "long been regarded as the most troublesome patient in the ward." He was experimentally started on lithium citrate on March 29, 1948, and within three weeks he had calmed to the point of appearing essentially normal. "As he had been ill so long and confined to a chronic ward," Cade wrote, "he found normal surroundings and liberty of movement strange at first," and because of this he was kept in the convalescent ward for an additional two months before he was discharged into his community, where "he was soon working happily at his old job."

Eventually, lithium became a mainstay of bipolar disorder treatment, although it was not until the 1970s that lithium took off as a treatment in the United States. Partly, this delay was due to the fact that since lithium is a naturally occurring element, it could not be patented, and therefore no drug company was enthusiastic to invest the money to undergo the testing required for FDA approval. Another reason for the delay was that lithium, like all other drug treatments, has side effects. Lithium's are particularly severe, and when dosed too high it can cause blurred vision, poor balance, and profound sedation—in some cases leading to coma and death.

Side Effects

The story of drug development in psychiatry is a series of unlikely and serendipitous discoveries. The bottom line for me as a clinician is that I now have quite a few arrows in my psychopharmacological quiver and I have to decide which ones to use when. While I have argued that this often amounts to guesswork, the fact is that the drugs usually do help to ease my patients' symptoms. Once I've chosen a medication, I have to deal with another inevitable quandary: side effects.

The issue of side effects of psychiatric medications has become politicized over the last several years. Scientologists, for example, who lambaste psychiatry as a "false science," consider the side effects of our medications to be a lethal attack on patients, whom are cast as our "victims." I have difficulty taking Scientologists seriously because they do not acknowledge the obvious effectiveness of psychiatric drugs. But beyond such fringe groups, there are others who make more rational claims. Legitimate psychiatrists such as David Healy of the University of Wales and Joseph Glenmullen of Harvard have written at length about the side effects of psychiatric drugs, particularly the SSRI antidepressants.[27]

The most common side effect of SSRIs is a deadening of patients' sexual lives. Both men and women experience a spectrum of problems, including lowered sex drive, a sense of numbness when performing sex, and an inability to achieve orgasm. In men, erectile dysfunction and delayed ejaculation are common. Just how common are these side effects? When SSRIs were first released, we had no idea there were problems at all. The official guide to medications, the PDR, initially reported that Prozac's rate of causing sexual dysfunction was only 1.9 percent, and several studies thereafter estimated a rate of about 10 percent for SSRIs in general.

These turned out to be wildly inaccurate estimates. The early studies assessed sexual side effects only by waiting for patients to bring the problem up spontaneously, which many were apparently reluctant to do. More recent studies, in which patients were asked specifically about the problem, have reported rates of sexual dysfunction ranging from about 20 percent for the non-SSRI medication Wellbutrin to rates as high as 70 percent for the SSRIs Celexa and Paxil.[28]

We still don't know why these medications cause sexual problems, although most researchers believe the problem is connected to the effects of serotonin. Viagra, along with its more recent cousins Levitra and Cialis, can counteract sexual problems to some extent, but they can only enhance erections and clitoral blood flow; they cannot improve that basic engine of sex, libido. Some of my patients find SSRIs so helpful that they gladly choose relief from depression over having a sex life, but others are less willing to make this trade-off. Complicating the issue are recent case reports of patients who continue to have sexual problems even after SSRIs have been discontinued.[29] Are we creating a world of blissful people who are asexual? It is a worrisome possibility.

Lack of sex is one thing; death is quite another. The most alarming potential side effect of antidepressants is the paradoxical possibility that they might *cause* suicidal thoughts—presumably the very thing they are designed to prevent. This possibility first entered the scientific literature in 1990, when the *American Journal of Psychiatry* published a case series of six patients ominously entitled "Emergence of Intense Suicidal Preoccupation During Fluoxetine Treatment."[30] The article described in detail five women and one man who had been treated with Prozac soon after it was introduced for problems ranging from depression to severe anxiety. Some of the patients had experienced suicidal ideas in the past, but when started on Prozac, they continuously fantasized about killing themselves in violent ways. One of the authors, Jonathan Cole, a senior and world-renowned Harvard psychiatrist, said of one patient that he'd "seen patients who were suicidal before but never anything quite like this." When taken off Prozac, the suicidal thoughts went away.

It was a controversial paper, because depression itself often leads to suicidal thoughts, with or without medications. Thus, if a depressed patient reports suicidal thoughts after starting an antidepressant, the underlying depression may well be the culprit rather than the pill. The only way to tell for certain is to compare rates of suicide in two groups of depressed patients who are randomly assigned to either antidepressants or placebo. If the suicide rates in both groups are the same, the depression is likely at fault. But if the rates are higher in the antidepressant group, the antidepressant itself must be the cause.

Under pressure from a concerned public, the FDA eventually analyzed the data from all the placebo-controlled studies that drugmakers had given them over the years. And they found something that was alarming. It appeared that antidepressants *can* cause suicidal thoughts, but only in the youngest patients—those in age from childhood to early adulthood. Children and adolescents who took SSRIs had a roughly 4 percent rate of suicidal thoughts or behaviors, while those taking placebo had a 2 percent rate.

This new data prompted the FDA to hold two public hearings in 2004 to decide what, if anything, to do about the information.[31]

My colleague David Fassler, a clinical professor of psychiatry at the University of Vermont, testified at the FDA hearing on behalf of the American Psychiatric Association. "The hearings took place in an emotionally charged environment," he recalled. "Parents testified, telling powerful and tragic stories about kids who had committed suicide."[32]

However, none of the children in the FDA clinical trials database had committed suicide (the parents delivered testimony about children who had been treated in regular clinical settings, rather than in research studies), so much of the discussion at the hearings revolved around the accuracy and significance of the 4 percent rate of suicidal thoughts. It was a statistical minefield, because this figure was derived from different drug companies' definitions of "suicidal thoughts" or "self-destructive behavior." In one case, for example, a child who hit himself in the head was classified as "suicidal." Other cases were clearer, but panel members still found the data confusing.

"Based on the data presented at the FDA hearings," said Fassler, "there was no evidence that these medications actually increase the risk of suicide in children and adolescents." Nonetheless, the FDA ultimately voted to require a warning on the labels of antidepressants about a possible risk of suicidal thoughts in children, a warning that was extended to patients up to age 24 in 2007.[33] The FDA's most recent data on all age groups was more reassuring, showing that antidepressants actually protect against suicide in adults and the elderly.[34]

Since these warnings, antidepressant use has gone down modestly in children, but not in adults.[35] There is a heated debate among psychiatrists about the effects of the FDA warning. Some have argued that it has lead to higher suicide rates,[36] but others have disagreed, pointing out that resolving this issue will likely take many years as we collect more data on drug prescriptions and rates of suicide.

Meanwhile, most psychiatrists, including myself, continue to prescribe antidepressants to all age groups, but we are now more inclined to warn patients about the possibility of increased suicidality as they first begin taking the pills, and to see them for follow-up visits more frequently. In my own practice, I have yet to see a patient who I was convinced became suicidal as a result of an antidepressant. Much more commonly, antidepressants make patients feel better, and I add psychotherapy to get at the root of patients' suicidality.

The bottom line is that when we prescribe drugs in abundance and with little understanding of how they work, unforeseen side effects are inevitable. We are beginning to understand the limitations of our medications, and I believe that over time, psychiatrists will become more cautious in their prescribing habits, and appropriately so.

Unfortunately, at the same time as we are trying to kick the habit of always reaching for the prescription pad, we are increasingly confronted by the juggernaut of pharmaceutical promotion. In this battle, our ignorance of drug mechanisms works against us. Since all the drugs within a therapeutic class seem equivalent, there is little scientific reason to choose one over another. And where there is a scientific vacuum, drug companies are happy to insert a marketing message and call it science. As a result, psychiatry has become a proving ground for outrageous manipulations of science in the service of profit. Many of the leaders of our field have allowed themselves to become paid puppets of the pharmaceutical industry. As we shall see in the next two chapters, psychiatry is in the midst of a crisis in ethics, and it is not clear if the profession will survive this crisis intact.

Chapter 5

How Companies Sell Psychiatrists on Their Drugs

In 1993, the FDA approved Neurontin for the treatment of epilepsy.[1] This should have been a cause for celebration at Warner-Lambert, the drug company that introduced it, but the celebration was muted. The FDA had downgraded the approval, saying that since Neurontin's data was not strong enough, the drug could only be used as an add-on drug for patients who had failed to respond to a primary epilepsy drug.

This limited indication was a problem for executives at Warner-Lambert, because it meant that Neurontin was unlikely to find its way onto doctors' prescription pads. The market for such adjunctive epilepsy drugs is small, and the company estimated that it could make no more than about $500 million over the drug's patented lifetime. That may seem like good money to you and me, but it is positively mediocre for drug companies, which define very successful drugs as those bringing in $1 billion or more in sales per *year*. Measured by this exalted standard, Neurontin was a turkey.

The executives, therefore, came up with a new marketing plan. A number of small studies and case series had shown that Neurontin might be effective for several other conditions, such as bipolar disorder, migraine headaches, neuropathic pain, and ADHD. The evidence was poor, and it did not meet the FDA's criteria for proof of effectiveness, but the executives decided to try to convince doctors to prescribe it for these disorders anyway. After all, doctors are free to prescribe medications for anything they want, even if there is no official FDA indication. This is called "off-label" prescribing.

Warner-Lambert was well aware, however, that it is illegal for drug companies to explicitly market their drugs for off-label uses. Nonetheless, according to a series of stories written by *New York Times* journalist Melody Peterson, such legal technicalities didn't seem to bother this ethically challenged company. Peterson interviewed David Franklin, a former Warner-Lambert employee-turned whistle blower, who detailed his former company's systematic off-label marketing campaign for Neurontin. Franklin recounted a meeting at which John Ford, a senior executive, exhorted reps to pitch Neurontin to doctors for a long list of disorders, none of them adequately researched. "That's where we need to be, holding their hand and whispering in their ear," Ford said, referring to the doctors, "Neurontin for pain, Neurontin for monotherapy, Neurontin for bipolar, Neurontin for everything." He went further, encouraging reps to get doctors to ramp the dose up higher than FDA's recommended maximum of 1,800 mg/day: "I don't want to hear that safety crap either," he said. "Have you tried Neurontin? Every one of you should take one just to see there is nothing. It's a great drug."

Warner-Lambert kept pushing the envelope of ethics to the point that it was eventually torn to shreds. According to Peterson's reporting, drug reps were explicitly instructed to not leave a paper trail: "Anything you write down can be audited. So don't write anything down," they were told by executives who were concerned about future lawsuits.

The company rewarded doctors who prescribed high amounts of Neurontin with free trips, dinners, or cash, essentially bribing doctors to use more of the drug.

The company hired marketing firms to ghost-write articles pushing Neurontin; physicians were paid $1,000 for nothing more than permission to be listed as authors. One memo from this marketing firm read "DRAFT COMPLETED. WE JUST NEED AN AUTHOR."

The company paid doctors to allow reps to read patient records and to shadow doctors during visits. In some cases, reps convinced doctors to prescribe Neurontin for off-label uses during these so-called preceptorships.

These sleazy techniques worked beautifully. The drug became a blockbuster, earning $2.7 billion in 2003 alone. Almost all of that income was from off-label uses; in 2004, experts estimated that 90 percent of Neurontin prescriptions were for disorders not approved by the FDA. Eventually, due partly to David Franklin's revelations, Pfizer (which had since bought Warner-Lambert) pleaded guilty to criminal charges and agreed to pay $430 million in fines—a pittance in comparison with the billions the drug was earning per year. For Pfizer, it was simply another business expense, and a fairly minor one at that.

Meanwhile, I saw my colleagues in psychiatry continuing to prescribe Neurontin for conditions such as bipolar disorder and anxiety disorders, even though the newest definitive studies found that it worked no better than placebo for either of these conditions. Apparently, doctors had been brainwashed so thoroughly by the Neurontin marketing machine that the data no longer mattered. They were prescribing the drug on autopilot.

Big Pharma was once a proud industry, a scientific crucible that created the first antibiotics, cardiac medications, and chemotherapeutics. But over the last fifteen years, the output of drug companies has gone into a steady decline. A congressional report published in 2007 found that from 1995 to 2004 (the last year for which they had complete figures) the number of novel drugs introduced dropped by 40 percent. They found that most "new" drugs during that time—68 percent—were actually "me-too" drugs, drugs with different names but with the same mechanism of action as older drugs.[2] Bemoaning this trend, Senator Ted Kennedy said, "the report shows that much drug industry research doesn't translate into real breakthroughs for patients."[3]

It is unclear exactly why the pipeline began to dry up, but in response, companies changed their business strategies. Marketing and sales divisions were beefed up. And marketing gradually morphed into something different, larger, all-pervasive, and, frankly, uglier than anything that had come before it.[4]

The new marketing strategies are not unique to psychiatry, but they have pervaded psychiatry more than other fields, for various reasons. With little scientific basis to choose one drug over another, psychiatrists are eager for guidance, and drug companies have been only too eager to comply. In order to provide prescribers with evidence to use their products, companies have brought their marketing departments front and center into the research business. When they have had trouble finding legitimate independent researchers to do test treatments, they have designed and funded those tests themselves. When they haven't been able to find academics to write up the results, they have hired ghostwriters, and then paid academics to simply put their names on the articles. And when, heaven forbid, they have conducted studies that haven't shown their drugs to be effective, they have slipped the studies into file drawers, hoping that nobody would ever find out they were conducted.

My own education in pharmaceutical marketing began during my second year of residency at Massachusetts General Hospital.

Suddenly, I noticed that Paxil bagels began appearing everywhere. I first saw them in the break room of the psychiatric emergency department, then in the conference room of the psychopharmacology clinic. There were platters of sesame bagels, poppyseed bagels, "everything" bagels, along with an assortment of cream cheeses, and a big container of Dunkin' Donuts coffee.

Nestling up by the bagels was an assortment of Paxil paraphernalia, usually pens and pads emblazoned with the Paxil logo. Often, Walter the Paxil rep, a burly, friendly man in a suit and tie, was sitting next to this cornucopia, eager to bend our ears about the particular "advantages" of Paxil.

I usually partook of his offerings, but I felt sorry for Walter, because soon after Paxil was approved in 1992, it was already developing the reputation among the residents as a dud. Our patients who took it often complained of sleepiness, weight gain, and sexual problems. Walter stood gamely by his product nonetheless, arguing that few people actually gained significant weight, that the sedation was actually an advantage for patients with insomnia, and that the sexual side effects were no worse than those caused by other SSRIs. And Paxil, Walter pointed out, was not only effective for depression, but also for the anxiety that usually accompanied the condition. "Don't forget Paxil for your anxious, depressed patients," he would remind us.

Deciding between Paxil and its archrivals Prozac and Zoloft was made difficult by the fact that the FDA doesn't require drug companies to do head-to-head studies. The bar for FDA approval is set rather low. Companies are required to furnish at least two studies showing that a drug is safe and is significantly better than a placebo pill. In many cases, a company will conduct several trials to ensure they can make the magic number of two. Forest Pharmaceuticals, for example, had to conduct five trials to get approval for Celexa as an antidepressant—in two of the studies the drug beat placebo, but in three others it did not.[5] Companies are allowed as many tries as they want, since the FDA doesn't count negative trials against them.

Companies rarely pay for head-to-head trials comparing their drug with a competitor, because most drugs within the same therapeutic class are so closely similar in their effects. And if a company can show that its drug is only as good as another drug, that rarely helps sales. If Paxil were found to be just as effective as Zoloft, then Walter would have been unable to subtly imply that it was *more* effective. It's much better to leave such questions unanswered, because then there is no inconvenient data to distract the doctor from a marketing pitch.

Although Paxil had the reputation as the high-side-effect SSRI, such was GlaxoSmithKline's marketing prowess that sales were unaffected. Walter and his counterparts were deployed to doctor's offices and hospitals throughout the nation, marketing the drug as being *the* SSRI to choose for anxious patients, and Paxil soon became a blockbuster. Years later, independent researchers conducted a thorough review of the research literature, and concluded that there was no evidence that Paxil outperformed any of the other SSRIs for those with anxiety.[6] But by then, this marketing message had been so thoroughly engrained in the minds of practitioners that the findings were largely ignored.

Walter became such a fixture in our department that in 1994 he earned himself a cameo role in the resident's skit at Mass General's yearly holiday party. In that skit, I played a psychiatry resident magically propelled one hundred years into the future, and the MGH Department of Psychiatry was portrayed as giving a single diagnosis to everyone—temporal lobe epilepsy—and Paxil had become the only medication the hospital prescribed. One of my classmates played the role of the chairman of the department, and in a dramatic denouement, this turned out to be none other than Walter the Paxil rep.

The skit, silly as it was, was prescient. Years later, the *New York Times* reported that in 2002 the MGH Child Psychiatry Department had solicited hundreds of thousands of dollars for a "Johnson & Johnson Center for the Study of Pediatric Psychopathology." Johnson & Johnson (owner of Janssen Pharmaceuticals) was marketing an antipsychotic drug for children, called Risperdal, and one of the publically stated aims of the center was to "move forward the commercial goals of J. & J."[7] A drug rep had not quite become chairman of the department, but a drug company was paying the rent.

Walter's gift of bagels was stingy compared to the drug industry's largesse in later years. In 1999, for example, I attended the annual meeting of the American Psychiatric Association, held in Washington, D.C. I shared a hotel room with three of my former classmates from Mass General. In the exhibit hall, we raced from one drug company display to another, collecting "swag" in spiffy APA canvas bags that were themselves sponsored by a drug company and decorated with its logo. We competed to see who could get the best stuff. My bag was soon weighed down with disposable cameras, textbooks, long-distance phone cards, mugs, clocks, and innumerable pens—all free of charge.

At the Janssen booth, I chatted with a rep about Risperdal, the antipsychotic that was making the company billions per year. He handed me an invitation to a company-sponsored party, urging me to attend. Curious, I rounded up my friends, and we showed up at the address listed. It was the Smithsonian Air and Space Museum, and Janssen had rented out the entire facility—all 160,000 square feet.

A live band was playing jazz on the ground floor. There was a second band upstairs. Several buffet tables and bars were set up amid the Apollo command modules and vintage planes, such as Charles Lindbergh's *Spirit of St. Louis*. We headed for the sushi table, stacked our plates with hamachi and California rolls, and moved on to one of the bars to choose from a selection of beers, wines, and martinis—all poured out by smiling staff. On one of the upper levels of the museum, Janssen had hired a team of photographers to take souvenir pictures, which they laminated onto refrigerator magnets. I still have that photo. In it, the four of us are smiling and lifting our wineglasses in a toast, and the Risperdal logo is positioned below us. We look deliriously happy—and why not? When had we ever been treated like such royalty?

Drug companies treat doctors like royalty because we hold the keys to their kingdom of riches. In the strange economic world of prescription drugs, as Senator Estes Kefauver once said, "He who buys does not order, and he who orders does not buy."[8] In this system neither the patient nor the doctor keeps track of how expensive new drugs are, because neither one foots the bill. As a doctor, I pay nothing when I write out a prescription, and my patients are responsible only for a minimal co-pay. There's no incentive to bargain hunt, and drug companies exploit this topsy-turvy situation by setting astronomical prices for their newest medications.

Drug companies defend their pricing by arguing that they spend vast sums on research and development on many drugs that never make it to market. Accordingly, they argue, they are forced to charge dearly for the few drugs that make it through the FDA in order to recoup their expenses. It's a reasonable-sounding argument, but it doesn't wash with the actual numbers. It is true that companies spend plenty on R & D—$30 billion in 2007 alone. But they spend twice as much on marketing—close to $60 billion in that same year. Some 90 percent of this marketing money is spent on sales activities directed toward physicians.[9]

Thus, rather than saying that drug companies are forced to charge high prices in order to develop new medications, a more accurate statement is that they must charge high prices to support a gigantic sales and marketing machine. Companies need so many salespeople and marketers because they are accustomed to making unusually high profits. Drug companies are consistently among the top three most profitable industries in the world. In 2002, according to Public Citizen, a nonprofit watchdog group, the combined profits of the top ten pharmaceutical companies in the Fortune 500 exceeded the combined profits of the other 490 companies *combined.*[10]

Psychiatric drugs in particular have been spectacular sellers for the pharmaceutical industry. In 2003, antidepressants were the single most profitable class of drugs for drug companies worldwide. In 2008, Eli Lilly's top two best sellers were psychiatric drugs: the antipsychotic Zyprexa brought in $4.7 billion/year, while the antidepressant Cymbalta grossed $2.7 billion—and sales were growing at a 60 percent annual clip.[11] Wyeth's best-selling drug is the antidepressant Effexor, with $3.8 billion in sales in 2007.[12] And Forest Laboratories' two top-selling drugs are also psychopharmacological: the antidepressant Lexapro (over $2 billion per year) and the Alzheimer's drug Namenda (about $800 million per year).[13]

This is why, once we hang up a shingle and start a practice, drug reps descend on us like hordes of locusts—if quite attractive, friendly, and well-dressed locusts. They rarely have degrees in medical fields, though they are given intensive training by the drug company in the advantages of their particular medications and in the disadvantages of the competitors. Mostly, drug reps are great salespeople, and their job is to figure out how to get the doctors in their sales territory to prescribe more of their product. Shahram Ahari, a former rep for Eli Lilly, summed up his duties succinctly in an article published in the journal *PLoS Medicine*: "It's my job to figure out what a physician's price is. For some it's dinner at the finest restaurants, for others it's enough convincing data to let them prescribe confidently and for others it's my attention and friendship . . . but at the most basic level, everything is for sale and everything is an exchange."[14]

It may be hard for people to imagine that drug reps can get us to prescribe a particular drug by simply giving us a meal or being nice to us. The process is subtle, but it happens all the time. To quote Ahari again: "Drug reps increase drug sales by influencing physicians, and they do so with finely titrated doses of friendship."

Valerie, for example, was my Ambien rep. Ambien, marketed by Sanofi-Aventis, was the first in a new category of sleeping pill, the "non-benzodiazepines." Standard sleeping pills, like Valium or Restoril, are benzodiazepines, and they work by latching onto brain receptors for a naturally occurring neurotransmitter called GABA. This latching on boosts GABA's effects, and GABA is unique because instead of activating neighboring neurons, it *inhibits* them. Thus, benzos enhance the quieting properties of GABA, and the result is a sensation of sleepiness and relaxation.

Ambien, Sonata, and Lunesta also bind to GABA receptors, but they are more selective in what part of the receptor they bind to. Because of this selectivity, non-benzos cause mainly sleepiness and less relaxation. This, in turn, makes them less addictive than benzos, which is their only genuine advantage.

I first met Valerie about a year before Ambien was slated to go off-patent. Sanofi had generated a new medication to replace it, Ambien CR (short for "Controlled Release"), and was marketing it as an improved version of Ambien. As is common when companies produce a slightly altered version of their old model, Sanofi had dropped all marketing efforts for Ambien, which only several months earlier had been the greatest gift to sleep since the Serta mattress. Paradoxically, Ambien was now the enemy, even more of a threat than other companies' products. Why? Because if Sanofi did not convince doctors to ditch Ambien and switch patients to Ambien CR soon, Ambien would go generic before this "conversion" could take place. Once Ambien went generic, its price would plummet, and insurance companies would pressure doctors to stick with older pills. Ambien CR would be left in the dust.

"This new formulation has two layers," explained Valerie. "The first layer has 60 percent of the medication, and it dissolves right after your patients take it, so they can get to sleep right away. Then the second layer dissolves gradually throughout the night, so patients can stay asleep."

"But is it any better than regular Ambien?" I asked.

"We have the plasma concentration here." She quickly pulled an article out of her briefcase and pointed out a graph in the paper. It was a comparison of the blood levels of Ambien CR with regular Ambien, based on a study done by Sanofi-Aventis in which subjects were given either one of the pills and then had their blood drawn every hour for the next eight hours. There were two overlapping curves, each shaped a bit like an elephant's head and trunk. Each of the two curves started with a big hump representing an initial peak in Ambien levels within two hours of ingestion, and then each tapered down through the next several hours, as each drug was gradually metabolized out of the bloodstream. The curves coincided up to the two-hour peak, after which the Ambien CR blood levels were somewhat higher.

"As you can see," she pointed out, "Ambien CR had a higher concentration later in the night than Ambien."

Looking at the small print, I could see that this was data from a small "phase 1" study, in which the drug was given to a small group of volunteers to measure how quickly it was metabolized. The study didn't include any measures of sleep. In fact, the volunteers were barely sleeping at all. They had to be awake throughout the study to have their blood sampled.

"Do you have any data comparing Ambien and Ambien CR on patients with sleep problems?" I asked. "This graph shows that the blood levels are a little higher with Ambien CR, but it doesn't tell me that real patients actually stay asleep any longer than when they take regular Ambien."

Valerie furrowed her brow, grimacing a bit. "I don't think we have any of those studies yet. But this plasma concentration data is pretty persuasive."

Not to me it wasn't. I had already seen the main Ambien CR studies and I was skeptical that this represented any great leap forward in sleeping pill science. Yes, the new pill looked promising on paper, and I had prescribed it to a few patients. Some of them said it worked well, some said it didn't put them to sleep as quickly as other pills, while others said that it worked too well as a sleeping pill, leaving them feeling groggy for several hours in the morning after waking up.

Valerie was persistent, visiting me as often as once a month, because she knew I wasn't prescribing very much Ambien CR. In fact, she knew exactly which sleeping pills I favored and which ones I ignored, down to the percentage of all pills I prescribed. Since the 1990s, such data has been offered for sale by pharmacies to drug companies. The drug companies pass it all on to their drug reps, who can access it from their laptops in the car before they visit a doctor.

Because of this practice, which is called "prescription data-mining," drug reps arrive at doctors' offices "armed and dangerous," according to Kathleen Slattery-Moschkau, a former rep for both Bristol-Myers Squibb and Johnson & Johnson. "They know what percentage of Prozac or Paxil a doctor prescribes," she said in an article in the *British Medical Journal*. "The doctor often doesn't know this and it gives [reps] an incredible advantage over the doctor."[15]

In my case, I was well aware that Valerie had this information, because four years previously, in 2002, I had spent a year giving talks for Wyeth, the drug company that markets Effexor. I would accompany Wyeth reps on their visits to doctors. They would provide the lunch, and I would give a mini-lecture on the virtues of Effexor. I eventually resigned from the speakers' bureau. I came to believe that I was deceiving doctors, and the experience gave me an unusual peek inside the prescription data-mining racket.[16]

Before I gave my talks, the drug reps would fax me prescribing information about particular doctors. One note, for example, informed me that the physician we'd be visiting that day was a "decile 6 doctor and is not prescribing any Effexor XR, so please tailor accordingly. There is also one more doc in the practice that we are not familiar with." The term "decile 6" is drug-rep jargon for a doctor who prescribes a lot of medications. The higher the "decile" (in a range from 1 to 10), the higher the prescription volume and the more potentially lucrative that doctor could be for the company. A note from another rep reminded me of a scene from *Mission: Impossible.* "Dr. Carlat: Our main target, Dr. S., is an internist. He spreads his usage among three antidepressants, Celexa, Zoloft, and Paxil, at about 25–30 percent each. He is currently using about 6 percent Effexor XR."

I also learned that drug reps have a list of slang terms for doctors, all based on how valuable they could be for the company. A "high writer" referred to a doctor who wrote many prescriptions, whereas a "low writer" wrote very few, and was unlikely to be worth visiting. A "spreader" wrote prescriptions equally among all medications in a particular class of drugs, and therefore would need a marketing pitch designed both to push the rep's drug and undermine the competition. A "no see him" was a doctor who refused to see reps at all, while a "sample grabber" didn't see reps but still requested that they drop off free samples of medications.

I assumed that Valerie saw me as a "high writer" who needed some consistent prodding to get my Ambien CR numbers up. One day she handed me a brochure entitled "Medical Textbook Program." It read: "Sanofi-Aventis is committed to your ongoing medical education.

Therefore, to assist you, we're offering the opportunity to select one of the following medical resources, compliments of Sanofi-Aventis."

I looked up from the brochure, and smiled. "This is great—thank you."

There were eleven options to choose from, and I ordered a small book on the basics of neuroscience. A few weeks later Valerie personally delivered my book—a modest paperback that sells at Borders for about $25. I thanked her, and Valerie left the office reminding me, "Don't forget about Ambien CR!"

Later that day, a patient came in complaining of insomnia. As I thought about the half dozen or so medications I could use, the image of Valerie and her gift popped into my mind. And I decided, "Why not try Valerie's drug for this patient?"

I was not consciously rewarding Valerie; it was more subtle than that. Gradually, Valerie had become a friend of sorts. Her face was familiar, she was always nice to my secretary, her presence was a brief reprieve from my busy days, and she had just given me a gift. It is a natural human desire to reciprocate when somebody does something nice for you. Conscious of it or not, I prescribed Ambien CR for this patient in order to return the favor.

As it happened, he didn't like the drug because of a hangover side effect that caused him a few difficult days at work. What if he had known that I had prescribed the drug to him as a favor to a drug rep? He would have been irate, and justifiably so. Patients like to think that we prescribe based on a careful review of the medical science, not because a likable rep just visited our office and handed us a book. But this is how salesmanship in the pharmaceutical industry works.

Gifts have become a central part of drug company marketing, so integral to the drug rep–physician relationship that the gifts are often not considered gifts. In a review of all the studies that had been published about the impact of drug company gifts on physician behavior, Dr. Ashley Wazana found that the practice is pervasive and highly effective.[17] It begins in medical school and residency. One study found that trainees meet with drug reps on the average of four times a month, and another study of medical residents found that they are receiving an average of six gifts per year from reps. These gifts are generally quite small, with an average per-gift value of $20, well below the AMA's current guidelines of a maximum value of $100 per gift.

Does the size of a gift to a doctor even matter? While formal studies of this issue have not been done, the story of the Hare Krishnas' business plan implies that tiny gifts, even when they are unwelcome, elicit a feeling of obligation to give back. Members of the religious cult used to frequent airports and would thrust trinkets into the hands of passers-by, saying, "This is my gift to you." Although the gifts were frequently unwanted and thrown away, the strategy encouraged people to make a small monetary donation, yielding enough income to make the group a wealthy organization. When drug reps give any gift, from a pen to a lunch to a luxury vacation, they are instilling a feeling of reciprocity in the doctor. It is natural to want to complete a gift exchange—in fact, social scientists theorize that social rules of reciprocity are an important glue holding societies together.[18] Valerie's gift of a $25 book was a single strand in her efforts to build a relationship based on giving back, and she got at least one prescription for Ambien CR out of the bargain.

While drug companies may be reluctant to do head-to-head studies of the effectiveness of their drugs versus competitor drugs, they are all too willing to conduct studies to disparage competing drugs. I became aware of this tactic when I ran across two journal articles focusing on the effectiveness of trazodone as a sleeping pill. Both were published in the widely read *Journal of Clinical Psychiatry*, both purported to be reviews of the evidence, and both reviews bashed the drug with the energy of a critic panning a lousy Broadway musical.

The studies piqued my interest because, despite Valerie's best efforts, I still commonly prescribed both trazodone and Restoril, two older pills that had always worked well for insomnia, and which cost just pennies per dose. Restoril is a benzodiazepine, a type of tranquilizer in the same drug class as Valium and Xanax, while trazodone is one of the older antidepressants. The effects of trazodone last longer than most other sleeping pills, and the drug has no addictive potential. Also, unlike Ambien, it rarely makes patients feel loopy and high. These qualities make it extremely popular among psychiatrists—it is one of the most widely prescribed sleeping pills in the United States.

Because I prescribed trazodone so much, I read the articles that were so critical of it carefully. Their points struck me as exaggerated and unfair. They said it lacked high-quality research data on its use as a hypnotic. But what they left unmentioned is that trazodone was approved almost thirty years ago as an antidepressant, and since it is no longer patented, no drug company stands to profit from doing large clinical trials.

They dusted off older studies highlighting some of trazodone's side effects, like cardiac arrhythmias or priapism (prolonged painful erections). But these side effects are extremely rare: Priapism occurs in one in five thousand men, and the incidence of cardiac arrhythmias is even lower. I had never seen either side effect in the hundreds of patients for whom I had prescribed it.

Why did these psychiatrists hate trazodone so much? Once I took a close look at the small print, it became clear. Each of the authors had worked as a consultant for drug companies that were marketing the newer sleeping pills, such as Ambien, Sonata, and Lunesta. In fact, one of the articles had apparently been written by employees of

Sepracor, maker of Lunesta, and the doctor may have been paid to be listed as the author.[19] Whether he had done any of the actual writing was unclear. Incensed by these sleazy practices, I wrote an op-ed piece for the *New York Times*, which generated an angry response from one of the academics I identified—but no denial of the facts as I laid them out.[20]

Apparently, executives at the drug companies had discovered a new marketing tactic: Pay doctors to trash your generic competitors. I imagined the following conversation at one of the companies:

Executive A: "Trazodone's a problem. It's eating into our business."

Executive B: "So what are we going to do about it?"

Executive A: "We need to get some anti-trazodone articles into the journals."

Executive B: "Brilliant. I know just the medical ghostwriter who can write the first draft. But we'll have to find an academic psychiatrist to put his name on it."

Executive A: "No problem. Dr. X is on our advisory board. He'll do it for a few thousand. Then we'll help him submit it to the journal. The journal will be happy to publish it, because we'll promise to order thousands of reprints so our reps can distribute them to psychiatrists in their territories."

While that conversation is a fantasy, drug companies' manipulation of the medical publishing world for marketing has been well-documented. For example, in 1999, as part of a lawsuit brought against Pfizer, it was revealed that the company had hired an agency called Current Medical Directions to write scientific papers about their antidepressant Zoloft. As detailed in an article later published in the *British Journal of Psychiatry*, in 1998, 1999, and 2000 the agency's ghostwriters prepared fifty-five articles and recruited high-profile psychiatrists as "authors."[21] Some of the articles were completed and ready for submission to journals well before a willing academic was located. In such cases, the documents initially listed the name of the author as "TBD"—"to be determined," and once willing prospects were located, they were paid an honorarium to affix their names to them.

The articles prepared by Current Medical Directions were published in the nation's top journals, including the *American Journal of Psychiatry* and the *Journal of the American Medical Association*. Only two of the fifty-five articles disclosed to readers that the alleged doctor-authors were paid by the agency or that medical writers were involved. Most astoundingly, these articles outnumbered those written in the old-fashioned way, comprising over half—57 percent—of all articles published about Zoloft in the entire medical literature from 1998 to 2000. Thus, for at least one antidepressant, the bulk of the medical literature was literally written by the drug company that manufactured the drug, which is about as glaring a manipulation of science as one can imagine.

Unsurprisingly, research sponsored by companies almost always produces positive results for the sponsor's drug. This has been documented in research on a vast array of treatments, including antidepressants, antipsychotics, birth control pills, arthritis medications, and drugs for Alzheimer's dementia. A meta-analysis of all such studies found that drug company–sponsored studies were four times more likely to produce a favorable outcome for the sponsor's drug than studies with other funders.[22] The whole process of pharmaceutical research reminds me of a quote from Otto von Bismarck: "Laws are like sausages, it is better not to see them being made."

But the story gets worse. Not only do drug companies control how so many studies are designed and written, they also routinely hide studies that don't look good for their drugs. While this practice, called "publication bias," has long been suspected, the vast scope of the technique was only uncovered in January of 2008, when an Oregon psychiatrist named Erick Turner and colleagues published an astonishing paper in the *New England Journal of Medicine*.[23]

Turner was uniquely suited to dig up this data because he used to work at the FDA reviewing psychiatric drug trials submitted by companies. In an interview, Turner told me that the idea for his study came to him partly because his psychiatrist colleagues seemed overly convinced of the effectiveness of antidepressants.

"People seem to view drug efficacy as a black-or-white phenomenon and, because these drugs were approved by the FDA, they must be effective, and that's that. This view gets reinforced when they look in medical journals and see nothing but positive study results," he said. "I would say they fail to beat placebo in 40 percent to 50 percent of clinical trials, and they would say, 'What are you talking about? I have never seen a negative study.'"[24] But Turner knew differently, because during his time at the FDA he had reviewed many clinical trials with negative results, and knew that many were never published.

He made it his personal project to try to find out exactly what percentage of these clinical trials were discreetly stuffed into a file drawer rather than published in a medical journal. It wasn't easy, because he no longer worked at the FDA, and therefore no longer had access to the submitted data. He and his colleagues spent hours searching the bowels of the FDA Web site, submitting requests through the Freedom of Information Act (FOIA), and contacting researchers who had previously gotten FDA data through FOIA requests.

Eventually, Turner and his colleagues tracked down the fate of all the research that had been submitted to the FDA about twelve newer antidepressants approved from 1987 to 2004. This included all the SSRIs, both of the dual reuptake inhibitors (Effexor and Cymbalta), and several other antidepressants, such as Wellbutrin, Remeron, and Serzone. These twelve drugs were approved on the basis of seventy-four clinical studies that the drug companies submitted to the FDA. Thirty-eight of the studies were positive, meaning that the antidepressant was significantly more effective than a placebo. Almost all of these (thirty-seven of thirty-eight) had been published in medical journals—no surprise there. However, thirty-six studies showed either negative or questionable results. Of these studies, twenty-two were never published, eleven were published in a way that inaccurately conveyed a positive outcome ("spun," if you will), and only three were published accurately as negative studies.

From the standpoint of a psychiatrist like me trying to figure out which drugs work, the bottom line was this: If I relied on the published medical literature for information (and what else can I rely on?), it would appear that 94 percent of all antidepressant trials are positive. But if I had access to all the suppressed data, I would see that the truth is that only about half—51 percent—of trials are positive. Turner called this the "dirty little secret" of the psychiatric world.

If there is only a fifty-fifty chance that an antidepressant drug study shows the drug to be effective, what does this mean for patients taking these drugs? Is everybody taking a placebo, and only fooling themselves into believing these drugs work? Fortunately, the implications of Turner's findings are not quite this dire, because the fact is that patients recruited into antidepressant studies are different from patients who arrive on the doorstep of my office. To get into a study, patients have to meet a series of criteria more exclusive than those of an Ivy League college.

Companies have found by experience that if they want to be sure their drug outperforms a placebo, they have to be very picky about which patients are allowed into the study. They want patients with "pure" depression, unblemished by messy problems such as alcohol use, anxiety problems, or bipolar disorder. Furthermore, because of reasonable worries about the safety of patients who might be assigned to a sugar pill, these studies exclude patients with suicidal thoughts. Other common exclusion criteria include an active medical illness, depression that is too mild, or conversely, depression that has lasted too long.

As I consider that list of exclusions, I have a hard time picturing a single one of my private practice patients who would qualify. Mark Zimmerman, a psychiatrist at Brown University, had this same thought, and he decided to test it. He identified 346 depressed patients who had shown up for treatment at Rhode Island Hospital's department of psychiatry. Then he pretended that each one was applying for a spot in a typical antidepressant research study, and applied each of the many exclusion criteria commonly used. Only twenty-nine out of the 346 patients, or 8.3 percent, would have gained entry into this exclusive club.[25] The only Ivy League college that matches this is Harvard, which had a 7.1 percent admission rate in 2008.[26]

To find such unusual patients, researchers who are funded by drug companies have to run a media blitz of newspaper and radio ads to encourage them to come out of the woodwork. The bottom line is that antidepressant research studies are not generalizable to real patients, meaning that few of their results, whether positive or negative, are reliable indicators of what would happen to *your* mood on antidepressants.

In fact, if you ask any psychiatrist in clinical practice, including me, whether antidepressants work for their patients, you will hear an unambiguous "yes." We see people getting better all the time. True, much of this response is undoubtedly due to the placebo effect, but it would be deceptive for me to prescribe a sugar pill to my patients while telling them that it is a real medication. So I am stuck with prescribing active psychotropic drugs in order to activate the placebo, with the main disadvantage being that such drugs have far more side effects.

Yes, I believe that psychiatric medications work, but this does not let the drug companies off the hook. In perpetrating deceptive marketing practices that manipulate the very science that doctors depend on to make treatment decisions, drug makers have betrayed us all.

Companies have told us that newer antidepressants with fancier neurochemical profiles are more effective than older medications, but unbiased studies funded by the NIMH have disputed this. They have tried to convince us that the newest and most expensive antipsychotics are an advance in science, when in reality they are no more effective than the first antipsychotic, Thorazine, and in some cases they cause more dangerous side effects. They have pushed the new sleeping pills by paying doctors to write pseudo-academic reviews bashing older medications that work as well and are sold at a fraction of the cost. In all these cases, when their studies have yielded findings at odds with their promotional needs, they have often locked the studies away in the file drawers, hiding crucial data from psychiatrists and patients.

Doctors are now fighting back. Beginning in 2004, the International Committee of Medical Journal Editors announced an ingenious plan to prevent companies from hiding negative findings.[27] They set up an online registry (at www.clinicaltrials.gov) where drug companies are expected to post information about all of their studies, regardless of the anticipated outcome. Any study that was not publicized ahead of time will not even be considered for publication in the top journals. The system appears to be working, as there are currently over eighty-two thousand trials registered.

There are other reforms in the works as well. The system of prescription data-mining is under serious attack, with eighteen states considering laws to ban the practice in 2008.[28] New Hampshire passed such a law in 2007, and in 2008 successfully fought off the efforts of industry attorneys to overturn the new ban.[29]

The pharmaceutical industry itself is also taking some initiative. In 2008, they strengthened the code of conduct for pharmaceutical reps, banning small gifts (Valerie's book is now off limits) and limiting the kinds of meals reps can buy for doctors.[30]

These are positive developments, but there is another type of pharmaceutical representative whose actions remain completely unregulated. These reps have unfettered access to the top academics of all fields of medicine, are invited by medical societies to give keynote addresses, routinely publish articles in the best journals, and offer advice about medications that is accepted as gospel by doctors everywhere.

These reps have medical degrees, and some have become millionaires by taking fat payments from drug companies. These are the hired guns of medicine, and they are the subject of the next chapter.

Chapter 6

The Hired Guns

The labels vary. Hired guns, thought leaders, key opinion leaders, drug speakers—even, to the practice's worst critics, drug whores. They all refer to physicians or other health professionals who join the speakers' bureaus of drug companies.

Most doctors who join speakers' bureaus do not sign up with the intention of becoming corrupt. They intend to speak honestly about the company's product, and to make some good money along the way. The corruption, almost inevitably, comes later.

In this chapter I'll detail my own experience being a hired gun, and then outline the sad tale of how the major figures in psychiatry allowed themselves, too, to be bought out by drug companies. While physicians in all specialties put themselves out for hire to the drug companies, psychiatrists consistently top the list.[1]

In the fall of 2001, a district manager for Wyeth Pharmaceuticals, which markets the antidepressant Effexor, asked me if I'd like to speak for the company.[2] I was immediately flattered, and when he mentioned some figures, I became positively intrigued. He offered $750 to give brief talks to primary care doctors in the area. I was making about $130/hour seeing patients in my private practice. Giving a single lunchtime talk would be the financial equivalent of most of a day's work, without the hassles of dealing with managed care companies.

Beyond the financial benefits, there would be the ego satisfaction of being considered an expert. Finally, the manager dangled another carrot—I would be flown by the company to a speaker's training meeting in New York City, where I would listen to talks from some of the biggest names in the field.

A couple of months later, my wife and I flew down to Manhattan and checked into a luxurious midtown hotel for what Wyeth termed a "faculty development conference." At the reception desk, when I gave my name, the attendant handed me a folder containing the schedule of talks, an invitation to various dinners and receptions, and two tickets to a Broadway musical. "Enjoy your stay, doctor," she said.

The next morning, the conference began. On the agenda were talks from some of the most esteemed academics in the field, authors of hundreds of articles in the major psychiatric journals. The first speaker, Michael Thase, of the University of Pittsburgh, was one of the most well-known and well-respected psychiatrists in the United States. He cut a captivating figure onstage: tall and slim, dynamic, incredibly articulate, and a master of the research craft.

Thase reviewed his own research showing that Effexor was apparently more effective than SSRI antidepressants such as Prozac and Paxil. According to his summary of eight clinical trials, Effexor caused a 45 percent remission rate in patients in contrast to the SSRI rate of 35 percent and the placebo rate of 25 percent.[3] If these numbers held up, it would be the first time one antidepressant was shown to be more effective than any other. No longer would psychiatrists have to rely on a combination of guesswork and gut feeling in choosing antidepressants for a patient. If Effexor was truly more effective than SSRIs, it would naturally become the drug of first choice in depression.

But I noticed immediately that Thase chose what was at that time an unusual measure of antidepressant improvement: "remission," rather than the more standard measure, "response." In clinical antidepressant trials, a "response" is defined as a 50 percent improvement in depressive symptoms, while "remission" is defined as "complete" recovery. Describing results in terms of remission made it hard for me to compare the Effexor data with other antidepressants in current use.

Did Thase choose to emphasize remission because he truly believed it was the most meaningful outcome by which to compare drugs? Or was it because using remission enhanced Effexor's apparent advantage over competing drugs? It was a troubling question. But it is the kind of question that is inevitable when a speaker is being paid big money by a company that stands to benefit from the information.

Jerome Kassirer, former editor of the *New England Journal of Medicine*, once described to me the problems inherent in listening well to a hired gun: "The reader or the listener has tremendous difficulty in interpreting the information when you know somebody has a financial conflict. You don't know whether they are being completely and totally objective, whether they are in some subliminal way biased by their financial connection, or whether it is completely intentional, whether they are doing it because they know that they will be in better favor with the company."[4]

The next speaker, Norman Sussman of New York University, went through the official slides that the company expected us to use during our own future talks. As he clicked through the Effexor Power Point presentation, he suggested ways for us to describe the data in our own future talks. For example, he showed us a slide defining the concept of remission. "Is the patient doing everything they were doing before they got depressed?" he asked. "Are they doing it even better? That's remission."

When it came to side effects, Effexor's greatest liability was that it could cause hypertension, a side effect not shared by SSRIs. Sussman showed us some data from the clinical trials indicating that, at lower doses, about 3 percent of patients taking Effexor had hypertension as compared with about 2 percent of patients assigned to a placebo. There was only a 1 percent difference between Effexor and placebo, he commented, and pointed out that treating high blood pressure might be a small price to pay for relief from depression.

It was an accurate reading of the data, and at the time I found it a convincing defense of Effexor's safety. As I look back at my notes now, however, I notice that another way of describing the same numbers would have been to say that Effexor leads to a 50 percent greater rate of hypertension than a placebo. Framed this way, Effexor looks more hazardous.

And so it went for the rest of the afternoon.

Was I swallowing the message whole? Certainly not. I knew that this was hardly impartial medical education, and that we were being fed a marketing line. But when you are treated like the anointed, wined and dined in Manhattan, and placed among the leaders in the field, you inevitably put some of your critical faculties on hold. I was truly impressed with Effexor's remission numbers, and like any physician, I was hopeful that something new and different had been introduced to my quiver of therapeutic options.

At the end of the meeting, we were all handed envelopes. I tore mine open and pulled out a check made out to me for $750. I gazed at it for a while before folding it in half and putting it in my wallet. Wyeth had already paid for a hundred psychiatrists to fly to Manhattan, to stay for two nights in a nice hotel, to enjoy meals and a choice of several Broadway shows, and now every participant was getting a bonus.

That evening, as my wife and I sank into our seats at Lincoln Center waiting for the show, I realized that with this much money being invested in me, there were going to be some significant expectations of a return. The question was whether I could deliver for the company without corrupting myself in the process. I would soon find out what kind of "medical education" I was expected to provide.

The practice of hiring physicians to give sales talks has become an integral part of the marketing strategy of all drug companies. According to a survey by Eric Campbell and colleagues, from 2003 to 2004 at least 25 percent of all doctors in the United States received drug money for lecturing to physicians or for helping to market drugs in other ways.[5] That works out to about two hundred thousand doctors. Amazingly, this is double the number of drug reps in the United States, which is estimated at nearly one hundred thousand, though this number is steadily dropping.[6]

Companies prefer to use the euphemistic term "key opinion leaders" (abbreviated as "KOLs") to describe physicians hired to do promotional talks. One former drug rep, Kimberly Elliott, who was once a handler for KOLs for several U.S. drug companies, described the functions of these physicians bluntly: "Key opinion leaders were salespeople for us, and we would routinely measure the return on our investment, by tracking prescriptions before and after their presentations." She added: "If that speaker didn't make the impact the company was looking for, then you wouldn't invite them back."[7]

Her assessment jibes with my own experiences. When I first joined the Wyeth speakers' bureau, I was scheduled infrequently, to give the reps a chance to watch me and see how I performed. Once they sized me up, they would share their evaluations with other reps in their territory. I was apparently doing a good job of "selling" Effexor, because soon I was invited to give talks weekly. I never did find out if the reps actually tracked prescriptions after my presentations, though they certainly had the technology to do so, since Wyeth, like all companies, purchased information about doctors' prescribing habits from local pharmacies.

From court records, we know that at least one other drug company—Merck Pharmaceuticals—did financially track the payoff from doctors' talks. As reported in the *Wall Street Journal*, Merck measured how many prescriptions of its ill-fated painkiller Vioxx were written by doctors after they listened to a physician speaker hired by the company.[8] Doctors who attended a lecture by another doctor wrote an additional $623.55 worth of prescriptions for Vioxx over a twelve-month period compared with doctors who didn't attend. By comparison, doctors meeting with drug reps increased their prescriptions by only $165.87.

Not content with the raw numbers, Merck then calculated their return on investment, after subtracting out the extra cost of hiring a doctor to speak. The return was 3.66 times the investment for the doctor talks versus 1.96 for the drug rep meetings. Not surprisingly, Merck made extensive use of hired guns in its marketing of Vioxx, which was marketed as a low-side-effect alternative to ibuprofen for arthritis pain. While effective in the short run, this strategy backfired on the company when serious cardiac side effects of the drug were revealed. According to an FDA researcher, Vioxx was responsible for up to 140,000 cases of serious heart disease before it was pulled from the market.

Drug companies expect hired guns to toe a fine line. They are expected to push the company's product, but not so blatantly that they will lose their credibility. Ultimately, though, the hired guns learn that they are, indeed, hired to accomplish something specific. The renowned psychiatrist Giovanni Fava put the matter succinctly in the pages of the *British Medical Journal*: "The game is clear: to get as close as possible to universal prescribing of a drug by manipulating evidence and withholding data."[9]

I didn't begin my career as a hired gun with the intention of selling doctors on Effexor. I saw my role as an expert consultant to the primary care doctors who were my most frequent audience. I wanted to teach them how to diagnose depression, how to treat it, and when to refer to a psychiatrist.

My very first talk introduced me to the realities of my new job rather quickly. After a forty-five-minute drive to a doctor's office in New Hampshire, I found the waiting room and walked up to the receptionist. She slid the glass partition open and asked if I had an appointment.

"Actually, I'm here to meet with the doctor."

"Oh, O.K. And is that a scheduled appointment?"

"I'm here to give a talk."

A light went on. "Oh, are you part of the drug lunch?"

There was no dressing it up. I was now classified as one facet of a lunch helping to pitch a drug, a convincing sidekick to help the sales rep. Eventually, with an internal wince, I began to introduce myself as "Dr. Carlat, here for the Wyeth lunch."

The drug rep who arranged the lunch was always there, usually an attractive, vivacious woman with platters of gourmet sandwiches in tow. Hungry doctors and their staff of nurses and receptionists would filter into the lunch room, grateful for free food.

I would pass out a handout summarizing some key points and start talking. I've never been a natural public speaker, and was nervous the first few times, but these casual lunchroom settings suited me. As I became more comfortable, I enjoyed and looked forward to the occasions.

When I started giving talks, I tried to give equal coverage to all the possible antidepressants fairly equally, but I was increasingly mindful that the reps were hanging on my every word. None of them told me what to say, but I learned plenty from their body language. They became animated when I talked about Effexor, and their eyes dulled over when I mentioned competitors. I felt my behavior being gradually shaped through positive reinforcement, like a child who learns to say "please" and "thank you" from their parents' smiles.

The drug reps were my employers. It was because of them that I was receiving an unprecedented, magical stream of $750 checks. I wanted to make them happy. So I spent more time talking about Effexor and less time on Prozac, Zoloft, and Celexa. I began to dwell on Thase's study showing that Effexor was apparently more effective than SSRIs. I sped through negative aspects of the drug quickly. After these talks, the reps began smiling more broadly, slapping me on the back, praising me for having done such a good job.

It took a very different display of emotion, this time from a doctor, for me to realize just how corrupted I had become.

I was speaking to a group of psychiatrists, and I was launching into what was always the trickiest part of my presentation, when I had to discuss some of Effexor's side effects, the worst of which is elevated blood pressure. This is where the ethics of a hired gun are most tested. How honest should I be? Should I keep strictly to the party line? If I had negative experiences with a drug in my practice, should I discuss them or simply remain silent about them?

Referring to a large study paid for by Wyeth,[10] I told the group that patients are liable to develop hypertension only if they are taking Effexor at high doses of more than 300 milligrams per day.

"Really?" one psychiatrist in the room said. "I've seen hypertension at lower doses in my patients."

"I suppose it can happen," I replied, "but it's rare at doses that are commonly used for depression."

He looked at me, frowned, and shook his head. "That hasn't been my experience."

I reached into my folder where I kept some of the key Effexor studies in case such questions arose.

According to the Wyeth-funded study of 3,744 patients, the rate of high blood pressure was 2.2 percent in the placebo group and 2.9 percent in the group of patients who had taken daily doses of Effexor no larger than 300 milligrams. Patients taking more than 300 milligrams had a 9 percent risk of hypertension. As I went through the numbers with the doctor, however, I felt unsettled. I started talking faster, a sure sign of nervousness for me.

I was lying. Not the kind of bald-faced lie that gets you sued or causes your reputation to go down the tubes. It was a more sophisticated, high-class lie, what might more charitably be called "spin."

Driving home, going over the talk in my mind, I knew that I had reported the data exactly as they were reported in the paper. But I had not talked about the limitations of the data. I had not, for example, mentioned that if you focused specifically on patients taking between 200 and 300 milligrams per day, a commonly prescribed dosage range, you found a 3.7 percent incidence of hypertension. While this was not a statistically significant higher rate than the placebo, it still hinted that such moderate doses could, indeed, cause hypertension. Nor had I mentioned the fact that since the data were derived from placebo-controlled clinical trials, the patients were probably not representative of the patients seen in most real practices. Patients who are very old or who have significant medical problems are excluded from such studies. But real-world patients may well be at higher risk to develop hypertension on Effexor.

I realized that in this and in my other Effexor talks, I had been blithely minimizing the hypertension risks, conveniently overlooking the fact that hypertension is a dangerous condition and not one to be trifled with. Why, I began to wonder, would anyone prescribe an antidepressant that could cause hypertension when there were many other alternatives? And why wasn't I asking this obvious question out loud during my talks?

That psychiatrist's frown stayed with me—a mixture of skepticism and contempt. I wondered if he saw me for what I feared I had become—a drug rep with an MD. I realized that the money was affecting my critical judgment. I was willing to dance around the truth in order to make the drug reps happy. The money was so easy, and so good, that it had become an addiction. Soon enough, something would happen that would show me how morally repugnant my new job was, and I would quit in disgust.

I made $30,000 during my year of being a hired gun. I found out later that this was small change, and that some of my colleagues were making many times that amount, and were doing their best to hide it—in some cases breaking both federal and university rules.

This sordid tale began to unfold on May 10, 2007, when the *New York Times* published a front-page story profiling Anya Bailey, a teenager in Minnesota who had been diagnosed with an eating disorder when she was twelve.[11] Her psychiatrist at the University of Minnesota prescribed a medication that was an unusual choice: Risperdal, which is FDA approved for schizophrenia and bipolar disorder, but not for anorexia. Anya was prescribed the drug because one of its side effects is increased appetite, and her psychiatrist thought this might help her gain some needed weight.

It sounds reasonable. Unfortunately, two problems arose. The drug caused her to be sedated, and more alarmingly, caused a painful muscular knot in her back called dystonia. After a consultation at the Mayo Clinic, Anya came off Risperdal and was able to maintain a healthy weight without using drugs.

The case would have been a non-story if it hadn't been for the fact that Minnesota was the only state to require pharmaceutical companies to publicly disclose the money they pay doctors to do promotional talks. When the *Times* reporters delved into these records, they found that Dr. George M. Realmuto, the psychiatrist who oversaw Anya's care, had given talks for Johnson & Johnson, the company that markets Risperdal. Furthermore, the reporters discovered that between 1997 and 2005, more than a third of Minnesota's psychiatrists took money from drug-makers, including the last eight presidents of the Minnesota Psychiatric Society. Psychiatrists had collected more drug company money than physicians in any other specialties. One psychiatrist, Dr. Annette M. Smick, was paid more than $689,000 by drug makers from 1998 to 2004. She said she was doing so many sponsored talks that "it was hard for me to find time to see patients in my clinical practice."

But something more insidious than simply getting paid to give talks was apparently going on among Minnesota psychiatrists. Those psychiatrists who received the most money from companies that marketed antipsychotic drugs like Risperdal wrote three times as many prescriptions of these drugs for children as other doctors. The implication was that psychiatrists were allowing payments from drug companies to influence their prescribing decisions.

Many of the children who were prescribed antipsychotics had been diagnosed with bipolar disorder, which is a controversial diagnosis in this age group, an issue I will discuss at greater length in Chapter 7. Dr. Realmuto told the reporters that he had been convinced to prescribe antipsychotics to children in part because he had attended lectures by a researcher named Melissa DelBello. DelBello had been commissioned by AstraZeneca to do a study on the use of their antipsychotic Seroquel, and when the results were positive for the drug, the company hired her to give lectures about the treatment. But when asked how much she was paid by AstraZeneca for these talks, she declined to specify, saying "Trust me, I don't make very much."[12]

As it turned out, "much" is in the eye of the beholder.

Later, DelBello said she was misquoted, and that she was referring to the amount she was paid for a single talk. But the quote caught the attention of Senator Chuck Grassley, then the chairman of the Senate Finance Committee and a well-known watchdog of the pharmaceutical industry. He and one of his congressional investigators, Paul Thacker,[13] decided to find out exactly how much AstraZeneca had paid DelBello to disseminate the findings of the research favorable to their drug. Invoking the authority of the Senate, they obtained her disclosure forms from the University of Cincinnati. As it turned out, AstraZeneca had paid DelBello $100,000 in 2003 and $80,000 in 2004 for various consulting or speaking gigs. And this $180,000 was DelBello's income from only one drug company; she had also worked with seven other companies.

Outraged, Grassley discussed DelBello on the floor of the Senate. "Today," he said, "I am going to report on the actions of one physician to explain how industry payments to medical experts can affect medical practice."[14] After outlining DelBello's nondisclosures, he spoke in support of a law he cosponsored that would require all drug companies to reveal exactly how much money they pay doctors for marketing activities.

As Grassley put it in a subsequent interview, "The question is: Is Dr. 'X' prescribing a drug because he got a consulting fee or money from a particular organization that's connected with the production of that drug? I'm not making a judgment right or wrong, but if my doctor prescribes that drug, don't I have a right to know whether he could have a possible interest in pushing one drug versus the other because of some financial arrangement? If that information's out, you're probably going to have people act a little more ethically."

The DelBello case prompted Grassley to investigate the drug company income of several other high-profile psychiatrists, and quickly several very large dominos began tumbling down one after another. It was a sad spectacle for me to watch the leaders of our field suddenly mired in financial scandals. Grassley had discovered an epidemic of conflicts of interest along with efforts to hide them.

He started at Massachusetts General Hospital, where he found that three child psychiatrists—Joseph Biederman, Timothy Wilens, and Thomas Spencer—made a combined $4.2 million in personal income from drug companies over a seven-year period, but had disclosed only a small fraction to the university as required.[15] The problem here was not simply that these psychiatrists earned so much money—although the amounts were, indeed, astonishing. The more crucial issue was the fact that these psychiatrists were "double-dipping," because they were making millions as hired guns while at the same time receiving taxpayer money in the form of research grants from the National Institutes of Health (NIH).

NIH has a strict conflict-of-interest policy saying, essentially:

> We'll award you a grant from public money to do important medical research. But in return, we and the taxpayers want to be assured that you are using our money ethically. We don't want you to be making any side deals with companies that might have a vested interest in the results of your NIH research, because this money might influence how you conduct and interpret your studies. If you *do* cut any deals, we insist that you make no more than $10,000 per year, and that you fully disclose these arrangements to your university.

None of the Mass General researchers made the proper disclosures. It is unclear why. All three said in statements that they believed that they had complied with conflict-of-interest policies.[16] Perhaps they really believed that the millions of dollars they made in speaking and consulting income were unrelated to their NIH research grants. It seems unlikely. I suspect that they were embarrassed about the drug company money and were worried it would sully their reputations if disclosed. We may never know for sure.

Every time Senator Grassley turned around, he bumped into another millionaire psychiatrist with conflict-of-interest problems. At Stanford, he learned that Alan Schatzberg, the chairman of the department of psychiatry and the newly elected president of the American Psychiatric Association, controlled more than $4.8 million in stock in Corcept Therapeutics, a company he cofounded to test a drug called mifepristone for psychotic depression.[17] While there was nothing wrong with owning a stake in a drug company, Grassley found that Schatzberg was simultaneously the principal investigator of a huge NIH study—of the same drug, mifepristone. This meant that taxpayers were funding an academic to research a drug that, if successful, would turn him into an instant multimillionaire. Could any human being produce objective and unbiased research with that kind of financial incentive? Who would not be tempted to fudge the results slightly, or at least to exaggerate the significance of the findings?

The public relations team at Stanford embarrassed itself by stumbling through a series of bizarre defenses of this glaring conflict of interest. In a letter to Grassley, Stanford wrote that "we would like to underscore that Dr. Schatzberg has not been involved in managing or conducting any human subjects research involving mifepristone."[18]

Wait a minute. Schatzberg was the primary investigator of an NIH grant on the use of mifepristone for people with depression, and yet, according to Stanford, he was not managing the study? The journalist Ed Silverman of the blog Pharmalot.com asked in a headline, "Who's in charge?"[19] Grassley, on the Senate floor, was equally confused, pointing out that according to the NIH, the primary investigator is responsible for "day-to-day management of the project or program." He went on: "So, the question arises: How could Dr. Schatzberg monitor the research funded with his NIH grants if he was not involved closely in the study?"[20]

Ultimately, Stanford couldn't answer this thorny question, so they did what they should have done when the controversy first began: They removed Dr. Schatzberg from the grant completely, and appointed someone else as the principal investigator.[21]

But the crème de la crème of hired guns was yet to be outed. Charles Nemeroff, the chairman of psychiatry at Emory University, had for years been considered to be the most powerful and influential psychiatrist in the country, on the strength of a distinguished research career and personal charisma. In 2002, he was crowned the field's "boss of bosses" by a psychiatric journal.[22]

At Emory, Nemeroff was the principal investigator of a $3.9 million NIH grant to study several drugs by GlaxoSmithKline (GSK). At the same time, he was a permanent fixture on the speaker's bureau circuit, giving lectures to other psychiatrists on behalf of several pharmaceutical companies, including GSK. At one point, he had financial arrangements with 21 different companies simultaneously.[23]

For years, ethics officials at Emory were aware that Nemeroff was hardly a stickler when it came to disclosing his income from outside companies. A 2004 report by the Emory committee on conflicts of interest noted that he had committed "serious" violations of university policy. But the report was filed away, no action was taken, and Nemeroff continued to reap the riches of hidden industry relationships. In 2006, for example, he cowrote an article endorsing a controversial treatment device, the vagus nerve stimulator (VNS), without disclosing that he was on the advisory board of the device maker (Cyberonics).[24] The "clerical" mix-up, as he put it, seemed particularly inexcusable because Nemeroff was also the editor in chief of the journal in which the article was published. He was soon forced to resign that position.[25]

Eventually, the full extent of Nemeroff's entanglements was forced into the open by—who else?—Senator Grassley, who demanded that Nemeroff disclose records of all payments he had received from drug and device companies. In all, from 2000 to 2007, Nemeroff earned $2.8 million in personal income (in addition to his Emory salary) from consulting arrangements, but had failed to disclose at least $1.2 million. Grassley was particularly concerned about money he earned from GSK, whose drugs Nemeroff was studying with $3.9 million of taxpayer money. By regulation, Nemeroff was not allowed to earn more than $10,000 a year from GSK while he was principal investigator of the NIH grant.

According to the *New York Times*, Nemeroff signed a letter dated July 15, 2004, promising Emory that he would keep his earnings from GSK to less than $10,000 per year. But that same day, Nemeroff was flown by the company to the Four Seasons Resort in Jackson Hole, Wyoming, where he was earning $3,000 for a single talk, part of $170,000 in income he earned from the company that year—which was 17 times the figure that he had agreed to. In all, between 2000 and 2006, Nemeroff earned $960,000 from consulting and speaking for GSK, but reported only $35,000 on his university disclosure forms.

In response to the scandal, Emory removed Nemeroff as department chair, but kept him on as full professor and allowed him to reapply for more NIH grants within two years. Meanwhile, Nemeroff's public statement revealed an alarming lack of remorse: "I regret the failure of full disclosure on my part that has led me to the current situation. I believe that I was acting in good faith to comply with the rules as I understood them to be in effect at the time."[26]

Eventually, Nemeroff resigned from Emory altogether. Why? So that he could accept a new job, that of chairman of the psychiatry department at the University of Miami.[27] Hopefully, Miami will require that Dr. Nemeroff take an ethics boot camp before he assumes his duties.

After the frowning psychiatrist confronted me during my Effexor lecture, I decided that I would no longer tweak the truth during my talks. At my next Lunch and Learn, I was more circumspect in my endorsement of Effexor's efficacy. I pointed out to the doctors that the studies comparing Effexor with SSRIs had been short-term trials, often lasting no more than two months. It was possible that, given more time, SSRIs would catch up, wiping away the small advantage that Effexor appeared to have.

The reps were not smiling.

Several days later, the Wyeth district manager visited my office.

"My reps told me that you weren't as enthusiastic about our product at your last talk," he said, looking perplexed. "I told them that even Dr. Carlat can't hit a home run every time. Have you been sick?"

At that moment, I decided my career as an industry-sponsored speaker was over. The manager's message couldn't be clearer: I was being paid to enthusiastically endorse their drug. Once I stopped doing that, I was of little value to them, no matter how much "medical education" I provided.

In November 2007, five years after I had quit the speakers' circuit, I published an article about my experiences in the *New York Times Magazine*. I assumed it would be of some limited interest to physicians and to certain laypeople interested in medical ethics. As it turned out, I vastly underestimated the public's interest in the topic.

The *Times Magazine* is published in print version on Sunday, but articles are typically posted on the Web site the prior Thursday evening. By late Thursday, I was receiving e-mails at a rapid clip, at one point approaching one per minute. For three days in a row, the article was at the top of the *New York Times* "most e-mailed articles" list.

The comments were generally supportive, but several were angry, accusing me of being a hypocrite and a media hound. Over the next several months, various articles were published in professional journals, either referring to my article or the larger issue of doctors taking money from drug companies.

This topic, like most ethical issues, is not black-and-white. The bioethicist Paul Root Wolfe, when asked to comment on the practice of drug companies hiring doctors as speakers, said, "Best intentions go astray among the pressures of money and relationships. I don't think it's intrinsically unethical, but you are creating a situation in which it's very difficult to retain ethical integrity."[28]

I would agree with Dr. Wolfe. I assume that there are some company speakers out there who are able to always be completely honest about the sponsor's drug and still get hired for more talks. But those are highly unusual cases. As I have debated this issue with colleagues, I have encountered a number of defenses of hired guns. Here are the most common, along with my responses.

"I only speak for drugs I use and believe in." That's admirable. But what happens when a study is published showing that a competitor's drug works better? Or what happens when a new and dangerous side effect comes to light? The medical literature is vast and complicated. It is easy to "miss" an inconvenient new fact, and when there are financial incentives to do so, "missing" facts can easily turn into willfully ignoring them.

Dr. Howard Brody captures the moral elements of this danger well: "If one voluntarily occupies a position that exposes one to a system of pressures that increases risk of a later breach of professional obligation . . . then one could reasonably be held morally accountable for one's willingness [to do so]."[29] In accepting the money from Wyeth, I was inviting the temptation to deceive doctors. That in itself may have been the key ethical breach.

"I'm careful to disclose to my audience all my conflicts of interest so that they can more critically evaluate my presentation." Disclosure is a necessary first step, but it hardly prevents the speaker from slanting the talk to make the sponsor's drug look good. In fact, some research indicates that disclosure can make the listeners *less* vigilant, because they assume that anyone who is honest enough to disclose their conflicts is less likely to be biased.

"I get paid by different companies, so the biases cancel each other out." This might hold water if a given talk were sponsored simultaneously by multiple competing companies, but that is almost unheard of. Typically, one talk is sponsored by one company, and that company expects to get its money's worth of sales from the speaker.

"Professionals in other fields consult with and get financial perks from companies with which *they* do business—why shouldn't doctors?" Physicians need to be held to a higher standard. We are not selling cars, computers, or mutual funds. We are selling expertise related to the most precious commodity of all: health. Our patients rightfully expect that our decisions about their treatment are based purely on an objective reading of medical science and are not at all influenced by the promise of personal financial gain. Doctors who speak for drug companies and doctors who receive their medical education from such speakers stray dangerously away from this ideal.

Finally, why do psychiatrists consistently lead the pack of specialties when it comes to taking money from drug companies? It's not that we need the money more than others—psychiatrists make as much or more than pediatricians and family practitioners, neither of whom comes close to psychiatrists in the scope of industry collaboration.

I think it comes down to the unique problems of psychiatry as a field. Our diagnoses are subjective and expandable, and we have few rational reasons for choosing one treatment over another. This makes us ideal prey for marketers who are happy to provide us with a false sense of therapeutic certainty, as long as that certainty results in their drug being prescribed. Furthermore, psychiatrists feel inferior and less "medical" than other specialties. Working at high levels with drug companies gives us a sense of power and prestige that is otherwise missing.

But it is precisely our reputations and prestige that we are putting at greatest risk when we flock to drug companies to do their marketing for them. As psychiatrist E. Fuller Torrey, executive director of the Stanley Medical Research Institute, has said, "The price we pay for these kinds of revelations is credibility, and we just can't afford to lose any more of that in this field."[30]

As we will see in the next chapter, the price paid is sometimes much higher; paid in the form of an inflation in the diagnoses of conditions, such as ADHD and bipolar disorder, and in the prescription of medications that are not only unwarranted, but in fact may be quite harmful.

Chapter 7

A Frenzy of Diagnosis

On December 13, 2006, police responded to a 911 call from Carolyn Riley, a mother of three who lived in the Boston suburb of Hull. When they arrived, they found her daughter, four-year-old Rebecca Riley, dead on the floor next to her parents' bed.[1] The police at the scene found no evidence of foul play.

Carolyn Riley said later that the night before, she had given Rebecca a dose of clonidine, a medication prescribed by her psychiatrist, and had put her to bed. "Then I woke up to the alarm in the morning. And knelt down to wake her up. And there was no waking her up."

After an autopsy, the medical examiner concluded that the girl had died from "intoxication due to the combined effects" of several medications found in her bloodstream. Two of them, clonidine and Depakote (valproic acid), had been prescribed by her psychiatrist, Dr. Kayoko Kifuji, at Tufts University. Dr. Kifuji had diagnosed Rebecca with both ADHD and bipolar disorder when she was two and a half years old, and had prescribed those two medications, in addition to the antipsychotic Seroquel.

Although Dr. Kifuji voluntarily gave up her medical license

pending an investigation of Rebecca's death, the police eventually found evidence that the parents had intentionally overdosed Rebecca. Carolyn Riley had recently picked up two hundred extra pills of clonidine at a pharmacy, saying that she had lost an earlier prescription, and Rebecca's teachers and school nurse said she was lethargic, like a "floppy doll" during the days leading up to her death. An uncle also told investigators that Rebecca looked so ill that he urged that she be brought to a hospital, but that the parents refused. On top of this, Carolyn Riley had been investigated by the department of social services for child neglect, and Michael Riley had been accused of sexually molesting one of his stepdaughters.[2] Based on this and other evidence, police arrested both of the parents for first-degree murder, and as of this writing, they are in jail awaiting a trial.

Eventually, Dr. Kifuji was exonerated by a grand jury and her medical license was reinstated.[3]

But regardless of who was at fault, the case brought a larger issue to the attention of the world: How could any psychiatrist diagnose bipolar disorder and ADHD in a child who was barely out of her diapers? How could one determine that a two-and-a-half-year-old, still learning to talk, possessed the grandiose ideas and the euphoria seen in patients with mania, a condition normally not diagnosed until young adulthood? What was the basis for prescribing a cocktail of powerful drugs for a child so young?

Suddenly, the profession of psychiatry itself seemed to be on trial, and the psychiatrist who became the center of this controversy was not the prescribing physician, Dr. Kifuji, but Dr. Joseph Biederman at Massachusetts General Hospital. Biederman and his colleagues pioneered the practice of diagnosing bipolar disorder in toddlers. "They are by far the leading lights in terms of providing leadership in the treatment of children who have disorders such as bipolar," said Kifuji's lawyer. "Dr. Kifuji subscribes to the views of the Mass General team."[4]

Dr. Biederman and his MGH colleagues have long been controversial figures in the world of child psychiatry. The MGH Web site portrays Biederman as a savior, a tireless and passionate advocate for children's welfare and a trailblazer in research on pediatric bipolar disorder and attention deficit hyperactivity disorder (ADHD).[5] Dr. Biederman has, indeed, had a distinguished career. He is a full professor of psychiatry at Harvard Medical School and a prolific author and researcher. In 2005, he was ranked as the scientist with the most-cited research in the world on the topic of ADHD.[6] And according to a *Boston Globe* article, his patients swear by him, saying that despite his international fame and multiple responsibilities, he returns his patients' phone calls within minutes to provide needed advice.[7]

But soon after the Riley affair, the world saw a different side of Biederman. He was quoted as comparing his work on bipolar disorder to such scientific breakthroughs as the first vaccinations against diseases, which seemed to be quite a stretch. He also disparaged doctors who criticized his research by saying they "are not on the same level. We are not debating as to whether [a critic] likes brownies and I like hot dogs. In medicine and science, not all opinions are created equal."[8] And at a deposition, after he described his academic rank at Harvard as full professor, one of the attorneys asked, "What's after that?" "God," the doctor replied. "Did you say God?" asked the attorney, apparently stunned. "Yeah," responded Biederman.[9]

Given this streak of narcissism, it may not be surprising that Biederman has some enemies, and the Rebecca Riley case seemed to have brought them out of the woodwork. At a conference on bipolar disorder, Lawrence Diller, a noted behavioral pediatrician and author, announced that he "felt compelled to name Joseph Biederman . . . as morally culpable in providing the 'science' that allowed Rebecca to die." In a later op-ed piece in the *Boston Globe*, Diller reviewed some of Biederman's research, which he claimed led to a "modern epidemic" of bipolar disorder in kids.[10] In 1996, for example, Biederman published a paper reporting that nearly a quarter of the children he was treating for ADHD also met his criteria for bipolar disorder.[11] Up until then, bipolar disorder was almost unheard-of in younger children, but this study, published by such an influential figure, prompted psychiatrists throughout the country to dig for bipolar disorder in children. Bipolar disorder, with its suggestion of a hidden neurobiological cause, became a sexy disorder in child psychiatry.

To understand the implications of this shift, one has to understand the traditional definition of bipolar disorder. In the past, the diagnosis had been reserved for older teenagers and adults who had periods of depression interspersed with dramatic episodes of "mania," meaning at least a week of acting like, in the colorful words of one expert, a "gerbil on speed."[12]

My patient Myron, a financial analyst in his forties, experienced just the kind of onset that is typical. His wife noticed that his behavior had been changing dramatically over a couple of weeks. While he had always been interested in tracking his investments, he suddenly became much more enthusiastic, and she heard him talking loudly and rapidly on the phone to friends about an idea he had concocted for pooling large amounts of money for real estate investments. He seemed to be everywhere at once, making phone calls, setting up meetings, sharing too many drinks with too many people. He also apparently lost the need for sleep. Alarmed, his wife suggested that he needed help, but he refused, saying he felt "amazing." In fact, he told her, he had made an "apocalyptic decision" to cash in all of their retirement savings to invest in his new venture, in order to "bring us to the next level of wealth." Convinced that her husband was delusional, Sarah called the police, who brought him to a local emergency room. He was admitted to the psychiatric hospital, readily diagnosed with bipolar disorder, and started on lithium, and he has not had a similar episode since.

Myron had all the features of what we call classic mania—grandiosity, excessive energy, little need for sleep, racing speech and thoughts, and irresponsible spending. Occasionally, children with bipolar disorder show some of these same manic symptoms, but they can be tricky to interpret. For example, if a child has too much energy and talks too fast, a psychiatrist is more likely to call him hyper and impulsive and to diagnose ADHD.

Biederman and his team changed this by offering a new definition of mania that they felt was better suited for children. Their new defining mood for manic kids was *irritability*, even in the absence of euphoria or grandiosity. This irritability went beyond whining or tantrums. The bipolar diagnosis was reserved for kids with frequent tantrums that were particularly explosive and long-lasting, and which lacked reasonable triggers.[13]

Using irritability as a guide casts the net for a bipolar diagnosis quite broadly, and this led to more children getting the label. How many more? In 2007, psychiatrists and epidemiologists at Columbia Medical School did a study to answer this question and produced a shocking statistic. They found that the number of children and adolescents treated for bipolar disorder had skyrocketed from 1994 to 2003, not doubling, tripling, or even quadrupling—it rose fortyfold, or 8,000 percent.[14]

As striking as these figures are, they didn't really surprise me, given my experiences as a psychiatrist with a private practice. While I don't often treat young children, I noticed that many of the adolescents who came to me for a second opinion had recently been diagnosed with bipolar disorder by child psychiatrists and were prescribed some heavy-hitting medications, like the anticonvulsant Depakote or the antipsychotics Zyprexa and Risperdal. Their parents were frequently unhappy with the results of the medications, because the side effects of sedation and weight gain were more tangible than any beneficial results in mood. These kids typically had big-league behavior problems since grade school, including violent temper tantrums, disobeying authority figures, suicidal ideation, drug use, and stints in juvenile hall. A long list of diagnoses followed in their wake—oppositional defiant disorder, conduct disorder, learning disorders, personality disorders, ADHD—and, finally, the latest in the litany: bipolar disorder. It seemed to me that the bipolar label was simply an umbrella term being used to simplify a host of symptoms and life challenges. Simple is fine, if it leads to better understanding and treatment, but I wasn't convinced that it was.

Dr. Jennifer Harris, a child psychiatrist at the Harvard-affiliated Cambridge Hospital, wrote in a journal editorial that in her experience many "bipolar" children were wrongly diagnosed, and that the real issue was typically a tangle of social problems. But, she wrote, most psychiatrists either can't take—or don't want to take—the time needed to sort these issues out. "The enormity of the problems many children face makes the simplicity of a biological explanation tremendously appealing," wrote Harris in a journal editorial.[15]

Clearly, Rebecca Riley faced such enormous problems—poverty, a neglectful mother who had abused drugs, a father who may have sexually molested other family members. Her psychiatrist appeared to have wrapped these issues into a DSM-IV diagnosis and treated it with meds. In doing so, she was relying on the advice of the top experts in the field, such as Biederman. But can we trust the advice of researchers who depend on drug company funding for their clinical trials and who also pocket extra personal money in speaking fees from those same companies?

Every year, MGH's department of psychiatry receives millions of dollars in research funding, some from government, some from industry; in 2005, for example, they reported receiving $40 million in such research funds.[16] Over the years, Biederman's child psychopharmacology department has conducted a string of clinical trials of antipsychotics in children, usually funded by the companies that make them. The trials enroll a small number of children with bipolar disorder (around thirty) and test them on a given medication for a few weeks. The response rates are generally from 50 to 70 percent. The numbers sound impressive, and the results are rushed into the top journals. Psychiatrists read them, and, like Dr. Kifuji did, they try the medications on some of their most troubled pediatric patients.

The problem is that these are only preliminary studies, and prove little, because they include no comparison group of children taking a placebo sugar pill. They are "open-label" studies, which are relatively easy to conduct, and bring in a steady stream of industry money to the department. Later placebo-controlled trials sometimes confirm such early results, sometimes not. In the case of pediatric bipolar disorder, the larger trials for both Zyprexa and Risperdal have confirmed some of the results,[17] but side effects have been alarming. For example, children who took Zyprexa for three weeks gained an average of over eight pounds; the placebo group gained less than one pound.[18] Do the potential benefits justify the side effects? That is a fair question, but I don't want the drug companies that profit from these drugs involved in this risk/benefit discussion.

While Biederman would argue that the source of the funding affects neither his research results nor his educational talks, this is hard to believe, particularly in light of a *New York Times* revelation in 2008 that he had directly lobbied Johnson & Johnson, the maker of the antipsychotic Risperdal, to grant him money to start a pediatric research center at MGH.[19] J & J ultimately granted the center $700,000 in 2002. Internal company documents obtained by Senator Grassley revealed that one of the three stated aims of the center in its annual report was to "move forward the commercial goals of J & J." A J & J executive who was Biederman's main contact for the center's funding wrote in a company e-mail that "the rationale of this center is to generate and disseminate data supporting the use of risperidone in" children and adolescents.

In essence, the MGH department of child psychiatry had allowed itself to become a research factory for various drug companies that used the resulting publications to drive up the diagnosis and treatment (with their products) of pediatric bipolar disorder. The larger world of psychiatry began to take notice of this ethical problem. In September 2008, *Nature Neuroscience*, one of the world's most influential scientific journals, published an editorial entitled "Credibility Crisis in Pediatric Psychiatry."[20] The journal singled out Biederman as being at the center of an "ethical crisis" in child psychiatry. Biederman, they said, "did not adequately declare over a million dollars of income that he received from pharmaceutical companies as consulting fees, calling into question the credibility and impartiality that he brought to several of the trials he guided."

Ultimately, the questions regarding Joseph Biederman's use of industry money led Mass General to temporarily bar him from any industry-funded activities—whether research, consulting, or speaking. He can still perform research, consult with whomever he wants to, and give talks, as long as none of it is funded by a drug company. This, in itself, may gradually help psychiatry clarify the confusion about bipolar disorder. As the companies that stand to benefit from skyrocketing rates of diagnosis begin to recede from the conversation, perhaps we will once again develop trust in academia.

While Biederman and Mass General took plenty of heat about their research on bipolar disorder in children, there is, to my mind, an even larger scandal still lying dormant in the department. This is its role in encouraging the diagnosis of ADHD and in pushing amphetamine use in both children and adults.

Amphetamines have a long history in medicine, and the discovery that they are effective in treating what has come to be known as ADHD is another of the instances of serendipity so common in psychopharmacology. In the 1930s, Dr. Charles Bradley was the medical director of a small child psychiatric hospital in Pennsylvania. For new patients, his standard medical evaluation included a spinal tap. Excruciating headaches after this procedure were common, and were assumed to be caused by loss of spinal fluid through the hole left by the needle. Bradley sought some way to stimulate the body to produce more spinal fluid. The most potent stimulant available was Benzedrine, and Bradley tried giving this medication to some of the children before their spinal taps. While this did nothing to prevent headaches, it led to dramatic improvement in behavior and learning ability.[21] Though Bradley published his findings in 1937, the prescription of stimulants for ADHD did not become widespread until the introduction of Ritalin in the early 1960s.

Over the years, many drug companies have gotten into the lucrative ADHD market, and there are now upward of thirty different formulations of stimulants, including grape-flavored liquids and even a Ritalin patch. Such stimulants work well for both children and adults with ADHD, at least in the short term. Patients become more focused on whatever they are trying to do, and often perform better at school and work. But the benefits come at the cost of an array of side effects. Stimulants often cause poor appetite, insomnia, irritability, and, less commonly, paranoia. More alarmingly, they can cause sudden death in children or adults with preexisting cardiac problems,[22] and if taken for several years can cause growth stunting in children.[23] Like any powerful drug, the benefits and the risks of stimulants need to be balanced carefully before we make a decision to treat.

The explosion in diagnosis of kids with ADHD has, of course, been the subject of much controversy. In 2006, 2.5 million children were taking stimulants for ADHD; a jaw-dropping 10 percent of all ten-year-old boys in the United States were estimated to be swallowing Ritalin or an equivalent each day. But ADHD was no longer just a disorder of children—in the same year, 1.5 million adults were also taking stimulants, a figure that has likely grown since then.[24]

In terms of diagnostic controversy, adult ADHD is the mirror image of pediatric bipolar disorder. In bipolar disorder, the controversy revolves around whether we can accurately apply an adult diagnosis to children. In ADHD, the question is whether we can apply what has traditionally been a childhood diagnosis to adults. Drug companies have a significant stake in adult ADHD, because whereas the market for prescriptions in children might be close to the saturation point, the potential market for adults has a great deal of room to grow. Drug companies have realized that the prescription of stimulants to adults can become a lucrative income stream, and that they would be well served by convincing more psychiatrists to diagnose adult ADHD.

The diagnosis of ADHD, like so many other psychiatric diagnoses, is fluid and expandable. If you were a patient whom I was evaluating for the condition, I would ask you the following questions:

1. Do you often get distracted when you are trying to concentrate on something?
2. Do you often make careless mistakes?
3. Do you often zone out when someone is talking to you, not really listening to what they have to say?
4. Are you unorganized?
5. Do you tend to lose things?
6. Are you forgetful?
7. Are you easily distracted by things going on around you?
8. Do you tend not to finish projects that you start?

9. Do you tend to avoid doing things that require sustained concentration?

These assess the nine criteria listed in the DSM-IV for the "inattentive" variation of ADHD, which is the most common flavor of the disorder (the other two being "hyperactive-impulsive" and "combined"). If you have answered yes to six or more of these questions, and if you feel the symptoms interfere with your ability to function, you would probably get the diagnosis. And you would likely walk out of the office with a prescription for an amphetamine. It's as simple as that—alarmingly simple.

What about more objective tests, like computers and brain scans? Companies have been marketing computerized ADHD tests for years. These typically involve sitting in front of a computer screen watching letters flashing on the screen. In one variant, you hit the space bar after every letter except "y." You have to pay close attention in order to resist the impulse to hit the space bar every time, and those who are less successful are rated as more likely to have ADHD. It may sound like a reasonable diagnostic test, but when you actually scrutinize the validity data—as I once did for an issue of *The Carlat Psychiatry Report*—you find that these devices cannot differentiate ADHD from any of the dozens of other psychiatric conditions that also lead to concentration problems.[25] None of these tests are either FDA approved or accepted as valid by any medical organization.

The fact is that the diagnosis of ADHD is made on the basis of a brief interview, and it is a judgment call, based on the psychiatrist's best guess as to how your symptoms link up to the symptoms listed in the manual. In children, the diagnosis is often clear-cut. Owen, for example, was ten years old when his parents brought him in to see me. I knew he had problems immediately, because over the first sixty seconds he sat down and stood up four times in rapid succession. He then sprinted across my office and proceeded to dismember a Oaxacan giraffe carving sitting on my windowsill. It all happened so fast that his father could barely talk quickly enough to tell Owen to stop the various destructive things he was doing.

Once he dragged his son back over to my desk, he had to hold one of his hands to keep him from running. Owen was unperturbed. He seemed like a happy but very hyper kid. His father told me that he was disorganized at home, that his room was a mess, and that he lost everything that was not a major piece of furniture. He showed me a report card on which a teacher seconded the father's narration. She wrote that Owen blurted things out in class, couldn't complete his class work, and often forgot to turn in his assignments. This was ADHD, pure and simple. Owen responded spectacularly well to Ritalin.

But in adults, the diagnosis is rarely so easy. I'll give you two examples from my own practice of adults I diagnosed with ADHD. In the first case, the diagnosis was accurate; in the second case, it wasn't, and the patient suffered some quite troubling side effects.

Ronald was an advertising manager in his thirties, married, with two young children. When I first met him, he struck me as calm and deliberate—ADHD was the last thing on my mind. He told me he was always a good student, had graduated from an excellent college, and had been working as an account executive for an advertising firm in Boston for several years. He came to me at his wife's insistence. She was increasingly exasperated by his inability to listen to her, and by his disorganization around their house, especially on weekends.

I decided to ask Ronald more about his school years, and it turned out that, although he had earned A's and B's, he had always struggled to get his schoolwork done because of an inability to concentrate. He was intelligent enough to compensate for this handicap by working twice as hard as his classmates. "I was the one who stayed in the dorm room to finish assignments while my roommate was out partying," he said. He was generally successful at work, but this was also a struggle, and he had developed elaborate computerized checklists in order to remember to complete basic daily tasks. One of my standard ADHD questions for adults is "Are you able to sit down and read a book for an hour straight?" He smiled and shook his head. "That would be impossible for me."

Ronald responded well to stimulants and became one of those eternally grateful patients that all psychiatrists wish for.

But for every ADHD success story like Ronald, there is a Terry. A man in his forties, he first came to see me for marital problems. A few months earlier, his wife had admitted to an affair, but said it was over and that she was fully committed to the marriage. Terry struggled with whether he could trust her, and suffered a constant sense of anxiety and turmoil about this issue. I diagnosed him with an adjustment disorder with anxiety, and I saw him every other week or so for supportive psychotherapy and to prescribe a low-dose tranquilizer called Ativan. This helped both his anxiety and his sleep.

One day, Terry came in and said, "My brother made me promise to ask you if I have ADD." He had been distracted, disorganized, and unfocused for many months. I told him that these symptoms were probably caused by his continuing anxiety about his wife's fidelity. But since he pressed the issue, I went through my standard ADHD questions. He did, indeed, meet at least six of the nine diagnostic criteria. The writers of DSM-IV tried to safeguard against ADHD being too easily diagnosed in adults by adding a requirement that patients had some symptoms before age seven. I asked Terry if he recalled having these problems when he was in elementary school or high school. "I think so," he answered. "I didn't like school. I was always getting into trouble."

I knew that there are many reasons other than ADHD that kids dislike school and get into trouble, such as conflicts with parents, difficulties forming an identity, and boyfriend or girlfriend problems. I tried to disentangle such issues from ADHD by asking Terry about his family life as a kid. He recounted many problems, including a divorce, a custody battle, drinking in high school, and truancy. Did these problems lead to his difficulties with concentration, were they independent, or did his concentration problems lead to some of his social problems? Predictably, these were very hard questions to answer definitively.

Eventually, although I still had doubts about the diagnosis, I decided to try Terry on a stimulant to see if it would help. A week later, he felt better overall, and had more energy to do things. Although it wasn't clear that he was any less distractible, he felt strongly that the medication was helping, so we continued it. Over the next few weeks, he requested an increase in the dosage, and subsequently reported even better energy and mood. After two months, however, he began to report more anxiety about his wife. "I think she's been seeing that man again," he said. When I asked him why he thought so, he said she was acting "funny" and that she was leaving "messages" around the house, like pieces of paper folded in certain ways. Nor was it only his wife who was acting strangely around him, he said. He noticed that his brother had been having whispered exchanges with her. Several of his friends seemed to be talking about him behind his back.

I became concerned about Terry's rationality. While I had no doubt that his wife might, indeed, be unfaithful again, Terry was starting to sound paranoid, and even psychotic, and I knew that paranoia was a potential side effect of stimulants. I asked him to stop taking them, which he agreed to reluctantly, and soon after stopping the medication he stopped worrying about secret messages and whispered innuendos.

In retrospect, I feel certain that Terry did *not* have ADHD. He illustrates how difficult the diagnosis can be, partly because so many other factors can cause ADHD-like symptoms (in his case, anxiety) and partly because both the diagnosis—and the stimulant medication to treat it—have become enormously popular. As is true for most patients, Terry loved stimulants, because they made him feel high. It became difficult for me to judge. For some years after we stopped them, occasionally he would request another prescription.

"No, you can't take stimulants, they make you paranoid," I would say.

"But I felt so good taking them."

"That's because stimulants are speed—they get you high and they are addictive. And for you, they had very bad side effects."

Terry taught me how tricky the diagnosis of ADHD in adults can be, and also reaffirmed the potential dangers of stimulants. I have become more cautious about bestowing the diagnosis since then, and more mindful that some patients try to game the system by faking the ADHD symptom profile in order to get a prescription for stimulants. These drugs have become favorites among high-school and college students looking for a high or for chemical help when writing papers or studying for exams. As stimulant prescription rates have increased, so have the rates of stimulant abuse, and the consequences of that abuse. A recent study found that the number of calls to poison centers related to amphetamine abuse by teenagers shot up by 76 percent from 1998 to 2005.[26] Most of the calls were about a specific stimulant drug called Adderall, produced by Shire Pharmaceuticals. When it comes to Adderall, Shire, and the selling of adult ADHD, we can once again turn to Dr. Biederman and his MGH colleagues as key partners.

In 2006, I began receiving a series of unsolicited newsletters in my office about the importance of recognizing and treating adult ADHD.[27] They looked like academic publications, with names like "New Perspectives on Adult ADHD" and "Substance Use and

ADHD." Each one featured a different "Academic Council." There was an "Adult ADHD Academic Council," a "Substance Use Disorders and ADHD Academic Council," and so on.

The council members were mostly child psychiatry faculty at MGH. Joseph Biederman chaired the councils for two of the newsletters. Timothy Wilens chaired one. The fourth was not chaired by an MGH professor, but by NYU's Lenard Adler, whose disclosure listed financial arrangements with twelve pharmaceutical companies, including all the makers of ADHD medications. Five out of eight members of Adler's council were MGH faculty, including Biederman and Wilens.

Each of these newsletters came in a series of six to eight issues, and soon I had a stack of twenty-six newsletters. Although the articles had different titles, and each was attributed to a different author, they all contained the same rotating series of "facts":

(1) Adult ADHD is underdiagnosed;
(2) Adult ADHD is an awful disease, with many underrecognized consequences, such as car crashes, divorces, and job loss;
(3) Many patients who present with *depression* actually have ADHD, which you will find if you ask enough questions;
(4) Psychostimulants are extremely effective for adult ADHD;
(5) Finally, do not be concerned about stimulants leading to substance abuse, because new research indicates that they might actually *prevent* future substance abuse.

Looking at the bibliography, it was clear that many of the studies cited to support these premises were conducted by the MGH faculty with industry funding. And not surprisingly, the production, printing, and mailing of the newsletters were paid for by Shire Pharmaceuticals, the makers of Adderall and several other stimulants.

Beyond being free sources of information, each newsletter also offered something of more tangible value—the opportunity to earn free continuing medical education credit, or CME. In almost all states, doctors have to earn a minimum number of hours of CME credit per year in order to maintain their medical licenses. For a newsletter to offer such credit, the organization producing it must be accredited by a national organization—the Accreditation Council for Continuing Medical Education (ACCME)—and must claim that the information is accurate and unbiased, even if a drug company is paying the writers and doctors involved. I know the CME business well, since I publish a newsletter that has its own accreditation. I have never accepted drug company sponsorship, but I am in the minority; most CME companies actively solicit drug company sponsorship, with the result being that many of the CME courses and articles in medicine are actually subtle ads for the sponsor's drugs, disguised as education, which was a perfect description of these Shire newsletters.

Once I had digested all this information, I had to sit back and admire this Shire newsletter blitz as a superb marketing tactic. First, provide the top researchers in the country grants to prove a series of carefully selected research questions. Second, pay a publishing company to create newsletters with "academic councils" populated by the very academics who have done your research. Third, send the newsletters to every practicing psychiatrist in the country. Fourth, offer free CME credit in order to ensure that the doctors read the material closely enough to pass an exam at the end of the articles. Fifth, pay the same MGH researchers to hammer home the marketing points at fine Boston area restaurants—to which I began receiving a flurry of invitations.

This was an elaborate, expensive operation, but in 2006 Shire needed to do something, because its ADHD drug Adderall was about to outgrow its patent life. Once that happened, other companies would flood the market with generic versions of Adderall, forcing the price down. Shire was pinning its hopes on a new, extended-release version of Adderall, Adderall XR, which was being marketed as a more convenient once-a-day pill. Meanwhile, the company had produced two other stimulants, a Ritalin patch called Daytrana and another long-acting pill, Vyvanse. Both products were nearing FDA approval, and the company needed a big marketing campaign to keep the new products foremost in psychiatrists' minds as they considered which stimulant to prescribe. This series of "educational" newsletters was a major prong of their marketing campaign, and it eventually worked wonderfully. By the summer of 2007, Shire was the ADHD market leader, with 30 percent of all sales, and Adderall XR was making them close to $1 billion per year.[28]

Everybody seemed to win from Shire's newsletters. The company carved out a larger market share. The newsletter publisher (Haymarket Medical) got a generous grant from Shire to organize the campaign. Biederman and other psychiatrists earned an unknown sum of money for writing the articles (actually, it is likely that the articles were ghostwritten by Haymarket writers and that the faculty members were paid for reviewing drafts and listing their names as authors). The doctors who read the articles got free CME credit. Who loses in this scenario? Possibly the patients, some of whom end up wrongly diagnosed with ADHD and inappropriately medicated with the newest and most expensive stimulants.

Which brings us back to Dr. Larry Diller, the California pediatrician who had accused Biederman of pushing excessive diagnosis of bipolar disorder in children.

I met him for dinner at the 2006 APA annual meeting in Toronto. We were speaking together the next day at a symposium about excessive industry influence in psychiatry. Over Cajun fish, I asked him about stimulant use. Diller is one of the world's experts on the topic, having written two well-regarded books about it—*Running on Ritalin* and *The Last Normal Child*.[29]

"So," I asked between bites, "do we diagnose too much ADHD in the U.S.?"

With a melancholy smile, he said, "Danny, our culture is obsessed with performance, and our increasing use of stimulants reflects this obsession."

Over his three decades in practice, he said, he has realized that there are two types of kids with ADHD: "Those with severe ADHD, who definitely need stimulants, and those with what I call garden variety 'Tom Sawyer' ADHD."

"Tom Sawyer ADHD?" I put down my fork. "Now that's something you don't hear about every day."

"It refers to kids who are definitely struggling in school, have some problems with impulse control, have interests and talents that are not necessarily what the adults want, but when these kids are interested in something, they focus fine."

I thought about some of my teenage ADHD patients who had attention problems in school but could sustain a laser beam of focus on tasks they enjoyed, like playing video games.

"As I recall," I said, "both Tom and Huck focused well when it came to tasks like finding hidden treasure."

Diller gave me an impish grin. "There is no question in my mind that Tom Sawyer and Huck Finn would be taking medication today."

He tries to steer these milder ADHD patients away from medications, at least initially, and toward behavioral treatments. For example, one of the most effective nonmedication treatments is counseling parents about how to raise impulsive children. Interventions can be fairly simple, like having parents learn and use the "1-2-3 Magic" method of giving immediate consequences to their kids. Described by psychologist and author Thomas Phelan, the technique relies on the skillful use of counting and immediate consequences to shape children's behavior.[30]

While I loved Diller's concept of Tom Sawyer ADHD, back in the office I was confronted mainly by adults, not kids, who wanted stimulants. There is nobody to "1-2-3" adults, and at any rate, impulsivity is rarely as much of a problem for adults as lack of focus and fatigue.

Diller does prescribe stimulants for adults, but he is cautious about it, because he believes that the marketing activities of companies like Shire have led to what he calls the "fourth wave of physician-prescribed stimulant abuse" in the United States. In *The Last Normal Child*, he describes three previous waves of legal stimulant abuse in the United States—Benzedrine, prescribed for fatigue and narcolepsy, in the 1940s; amphetamine, prescribed for depression and weight loss, in the 1960s; and Dexedrine, prescribed as diet pills, in the 1970s. Adderall, another form of amphetamine, is currently the most prescribed stimulant in the United States, and it has overtaken Ritalin as the most abused stimulant on college campuses.[31]

"We love our stimulants in this country," he said.

Recently, a group of eminent neuroscientists and ethicists wrote a commentary in *Nature* arguing that people shouldn't have to get an ADHD diagnosis to get a prescription of stimulants, or the newer alertness drug Provigil, which they regard as "cognitive enhancers."[32] The commentary cited an informal poll showing that as many as one out of five scientists in the United States take Provigil or another stimulant on a regular basis to enhance their performance.[33] If this leads to better science, maybe it will lead to a better society, the editorialists argued, and concluded with a strange call to arms: "We call for a presumption that mentally competent adults should be able to engage in cognitive enhancement using drugs."

Ironically, this group of scientists, with absolutely no funding from drug companies, may succeed in expanding the market for stimulants beyond Shire's wildest imagination. If so, the company will no longer need to pay the best and brightest psychiatrists to convince patients that they have ADHD.

Diller points to what should be a serious concern: "Ritalin and I have been together for thirty-two years, I know it well, along with the other stimulants. You never know when a dabbler will become a drug abuser."

Wise words, but on the other hand, we never know when a potentially dangerous medication will be successful for a given patient, and psychiatrists hate to miss such opportunities. For all their drawbacks, the meds are often effective, and they are the tools at our disposal. Yes, I may rail against drug companies for encouraging us to diagnose more conditions and prescribe more medications, but without the companies I would have much less to offer my patients. And it is hard to blame them for doing what they need to do to maximize their profits—they are businesses, they have shareholders, and their attention is always focused on the bottom line.

I realize that this is their motivation, and while I prescribe plenty of stimulants, I also know how important it is to scrutinize their claims at every turn. When our most esteemed colleagues have essentially joined the marketing teams, it makes it that much harder for us to practice our craft responsibly. The resulting frenzy of psychiatric diagnoses has damaged the credibility of everyone in the field. Who, after hearing the stories of such behavior, can really trust any psychiatrist again?

Regaining that trust will take time, humility, and a willingness to admit the limits of our knowledge. Sometimes, we simply don't understand what we are doing, even as we are prescribing drugs that appear to help. It is only fair to let our patients know when we don't know.

Chapter 8

The Seductions of Technology

Michael looked up at me from the gurney, a resigned smile on his face. He was calmer than I imagine I would have been, considering that I was about to send twenty volts of electricity through his brain. I was administering electroconvulsive therapy (ECT) to Michael in the Anna Jaques Hospital's operating recovery room, working with an anesthesiologist and two nurses. I took my position at the head of Michael's bed, and one nurse started an IV line while the anesthesiologist lay out the sedating medications on a tray, a neat row of color-coded syringes.

"The IV is good, we're ready," announced the nurse.

I quickly got to work, wrapping a wide rubber band around Michael's head. "This might feel a little tight," I warned him. "Yes, I remember," Michael responded. Grabbing a tube of conducting gel, I squirted a little on my fingers and rubbed it onto the right side of Michael's temple. I then slid a round, flat metal disc of metal called a lead, about the size of a half-dollar coin, against his skin, just beneath the band. The lead was connected to a wire snaking out of the ECT machine, a device the size of a photocopier but studded with dials, switches, and knobs. It looked like a jetliner's cockpit on wheels.

After adjusting the settings, I signaled to the anesthesiologist that I was ready and placed an oxygen mask loosely on Michael's face. "Just breathe normally," I told him. "You'll be going to sleep soon."

The anesthesiologist took one of his syringes and plunged a strong sedative into the IV. It worked quickly—Michael's eyes began to flutter within thirty seconds and within a minute he was out cold.

"Michael?" I asked loudly. "Michael, are you awake?"

It was crucial to establish that he was in a deep sleep before the next phase. I nodded to the anesthesiologist, who took another syringe to the IV line, plunging it home. This was succinylcholine, something that I tell patients is a "muscle relaxant," but which actually causes temporary paralysis. Succinylcholine has transformed ECT from what once looked barbaric—picture Jack Nicholson flailing around on the table under Nurse Ratched's gaze in *One Flew over the Cuckoo's Nest*—into a well-controlled medical procedure like any other.

We waited for the succinylcholine to distribute throughout his bloodstream, and then I reached over to Michael's mouth and inserted a tooth guard. We were ready.

I reached for the second lead, another metal disk, but this one was attached to the end of an insulated paddle, through which another wire brought electricity from the ECT machine. I then rubbed the top of Michael's head with more conducting gel and pressed the lead down firmly through his hair. There were now two leads to complete the circuit: one on his right temple and the other on the crown of his scalp. The electricity would course through the handheld lead, go through his brain, and exit out of the temple lead.

"Treatment!" I called out, and pushed the red button.

After one or two seconds the machine had drawn the necessary voltage and let out a loud *beeeeeeep*, signaling that current was now flowing. Michael's jaw clenched, and I soon noticed a very fine tremor of his right arm. I looked at the brain wave tracing to confirm that he was having a seizure, and indeed, Michael's brain waves had transformed from neat regular peaks and troughs to a wild stallion pattern, indicating rhythmic activity of large swaths of the brain—in other words, a seizure.

Although the actual electrical current flowed for only a couple of seconds, the seizure it triggered went on for about forty-five seconds, after which his brain waves subsided into his regular pattern. In ECT, short seizures are curative; long seizures, which are rare, are problems.

The seizure over, I removed Michael's mouth guard, and five minutes after he had first been put to sleep, he opened his eyes and looked at my upside-down face. "Hello," I said. His eyes narrowed in confusion. "I'm Dr. Carlat, Michael, and you just had an ECT treatment."

During the first few minutes after ECT, patients are often disoriented, as the neurons gradually settle down from their electrical chaos. The nurse wheeled Michael into a recovery bay. An hour or so later, his wife arrived to drive him back home.

I had met Michael in the inpatient psychiatry unit at Anna Jaques a week earlier, where he had been admitted for depression and suicidal thoughts. His father, who was a hard drinker and had beaten him daily, was suicidal. Michael recalled finding him hanging by a rope one day and cutting him down just in time.

Michael had begun to take on many of his father's afflictions, minus the abusive temper. He drank heavily and suffered recurring suicidal depression. One day at work he walked into a storage closet, pulled up a chair, wrapped a noose around his neck, and attempted to kick the chair away, but the space was too small to accomplish this quickly. The noise alerted a coworker, who opened the closet door and saved his life.

Once he was hospitalized, I interviewed him and reviewed his extensive records. This was the latest of several hospitalizations over the years, and Michael had tried almost all the antidepressants but none were effective. Eventually, two years before I saw him, he had agreed to a course of ECT. A typical course involves treatments three times a week for three or four weeks. Like many patients, Michael had initially been reluctant, because of the potential side effect of memory loss, but once he had consented, the treatments had worked well for a time, causing minimal side effects. He was able to go back to work and to enjoy time with his wife and two college-age sons. But, as is often the case, the beneficial effects eventually petered out. He had relapsed within a year of both courses of treatment, and I met him during his second relapse.

This was in 1998, and I had just completed a fellowship in ECT at Columbia University with Harold Sackeim, where I had learned about the tumultuous history of this storied medical treatment. The idea for ECT came from the historical observation that when depressed people had convulsions, whether due to epilepsy or other causes, they often felt better afterward.[1] Surmising that seizures themselves might be curative, researchers looked for ways to purposefully trigger them in people. A Hungarian psychiatrist, Ladislav von Meduna, was the first to accomplish this rather dangerous procedure, when, in the 1930s, he found that injecting depressed patients with the chemical camphor could induce the episodes. He called this technique "convulsive therapy," and eventually switched from camphor to a cardiac stimulant called Metrazol. It worked fairly well, easing symptoms in about half of patients, but it did not reliably induce seizures—sometimes they didn't occur at all and other times they would be so severe as to be life threatening. It gained popularity, nonetheless, because the alternative in those days was no treatment at all.

But a safer method was needed, and the key advance was developed by a psychiatrist in Rome, Ugo Cerletti, in 1938. For some years, Cerletti and his colleagues had been studying the effects of seizures by using electricity to induce convulsions in dogs. When he learned of Dr. Meduna's new convulsive therapy technique, he shifted the focus of his work, trying variations in electrode placement and voltage to induce seizures in different animals, with the goal of finding a way to make this safe for humans. By 1938, Cerletti and his colleagues felt they were ready to test the new treatment, having built a primitive machine that was capable of delivering 80–100 volts of electricity.

The first patient ever to receive ECT was admitted to the University of Rome's clinic in April of that year after having been arrested by Roman police at the city's train station. He was a thirty-nine-year-old engineer from Milan who had been wandering around, hallucinating and saying that he was "telepathically influenced." Apparently, he was not depressed, but would probably have been given the modern diagnosis of schizophrenia. Cerletti interviewed the patient, who was amenable to trying ECT (the modern concept of "informed consent" had yet to be conceived). They shaved his head, placed the electrodes, and inserted a rubber tube between his teeth to prevent him from biting his tongue; then they conducted eighty volts into his brain for a fraction of a second. Not much happened. They cranked it up to ninety volts, and again there was not much response. The patient sat up, unperturbed, and made the bizarre comment (in Italian), "Look out! The first is pestiferous, the second mortiferous." Cerletti's assistant dialed the machine up to the maximum, one hundred volts. That did the trick—the patient immediately had a grand mal seizure, his whole body shaking rhythmically for forty-eight seconds. When he awoke, he had no memory of what had happened, and he appeared unharmed. He went on to have eleven more treatments while he was in the hospital and his delusions disappeared, allowing him to be discharged within a month.

The technique was soon introduced into the United States, where doctors added medications that transiently paralyzed patients' muscles in order to prevent spinal fractures, which was a potential complication of the seizures. By the late 1950s, ECT was considered to be the most effective treatment available for both depression and bipolar disorder.

But in the 1960s, various factors combined to create a growing anti-ECT movement. The Church of Scientology (founded in 1954), which became influential and was vocally opposed to ECT, charged that it caused brain damage. Ken Kesey's *One Flew over the Cuckoo's Nest*, published in 1962, portrayed ECT as "that filthy brain-murdering room that the black boys [the orderlies] call the 'Shock Shop.'"[2] The 1975 film version, with Jack Nicholson playing Randle P. McMurphy, a rebel who is converted into a drooling imbecile by ECT and a lobotomy, cemented a general view that the treatment caused more harm than good.

Since then, the treatment has been refined and made gentler by lowering the amount of electricity delivered and changing where on the scalp the leads are placed. After nearly disappearing from hospitals in the 1970s, it has become a fairly common psychiatric treatment. In 1999 the U.S. Surgeon General's office officially endorsed ECT, stating in a report that in all controlled trials of the technique, no alternative treatment had ever been shown to be better.[3] Now, about one hundred thousand patients in the United States receive the treatment yearly, and 1 million receive it worldwide.[4] It still has its naysayers, but they are fewer and less strident, and are apt to make more reasoned critiques, such as Juli Lawrence, a self-described "ECT survivor" who argues that psychiatrists minimize the cognitive side effects (often true, in my opinion) and that *forced* ECT is unethical (certainly true, though it almost never happens).[5]

The major problem with ECT is identical to the problem with psychiatric medication. While ECT works, we have no idea how or why. The seizure is probably the key antidepressant ingredient (rather than the initial jolt of electricity), but why a seizure, which causes neurons throughout the brain to fire simultaneously, would make people less sad remains a mystery. Some studies have suggested that the treatment increases levels of some neurotransmitters and that in laboratory animals it may cause cell growth in certain brain regions, such as the hippocampus.[6] But beyond this, we are completely in the dark. A recent description by a psychiatrist writing for a lay publication encapsulates the true level of knowledge about how it operates: "The seizure seems to reboot the emotional machinery of the brain, in the same way that pressing Ctrl-Alt-Delete on the computer can sometimes provide a fresh start when the digital computer brain is stuck."[7] Essentially, ECT somehow resets the brain, providing a neurological fresh start.

Not knowing how an effective treatment works does not mean that we should not use it, of course. But it does mean that we should be cautious about it, and more carefully weigh the risks of treatment, because the corollary of not knowing why a treatment works is not knowing why a treatment causes side effects. The main side effect of ECT is memory loss, usually a transient confusion that lasts no more than an hour after the seizure. There is a debate in the field about whether the memory loss is more extensive than this. Many patients forget events that happened during an entire three- or four-week course of treatment, and subjectively, about one-third of all patients who have received ECT complain of "persistent memory loss." But according to studies that assess patients' memories with standardized memory tests, cognitive scores actually improve over pretreatment scores within six months after treatment.[8]

Michael continued his ECT under my care, getting therapy every other day for a few weeks, and with each treatment his mood lifted more. He began to smile and laugh. He began looking forward to spending more time with his children and finishing carpentry projects around the house. After twelve treatments, we stopped, but as I had planned, we agreed to do monthly maintenance ECT in the hope it would prevent another relapse, and it worked. He went a couple of years without slipping back into depression. Eventually, though, he wanted to take a break from ECT.

"I'm tired of having to go to the hospital every month," he told me. "And I don't like the memory problems and the headaches."

He explained that he usually forgot everything that happened the day of his treatment, and beyond that, he felt that his memory for distant events was not as sharp as it used to be. His "headache" was more of a jaw ache, caused by biting down hard on the tooth guard during the seizure. We ended the monthly treatments, and for the past several years he has done well on medications alone (he had been on medications even during his maintenance treatments).

I stopped administering ECT a few years ago, in order to pursue a full-time private practice, and when I look back on my experiences in the surgical suite, I wonder why psychiatrists need to be present at all. My role was the pusher of buttons, the turner of dials, and the observer of brain waves. Meanwhile, the medical team did the grunt work—checking vital signs, putting in IV lines, administering medications. If something went wrong, and the patient had a cardiac arrhythmia or a drop in blood pressure, I moved out of the way, and let the specialists sweep in to administer emergency treatment. If I had tried to do this, I would likely have botched the job (few patients would want a psychiatrist to be in charge of antiarrhythmic medications such as IV lidocaine) and been sued for malpractice. Lab techs could easily take over my limited functions in the ECT suite, as long as they receive proper training and periodic recertification—similar to radiology techs, dental hygienists, and the many other physician extenders who are an integral part of medicine. Such "ECT techs" would likely not only bring the cost of ECT down a bit, but would make the treatment more accessible. In my region north of Boston, there is usually a long wait list to get scheduled for ECT, with the bottleneck being a dearth of psychiatrists who can offer the treatment.

But if we left ECT to techs, we would lose the only technical procedure that we can call our own. This would be another insult to our sense of being part of the community of physicians. Meanwhile, the device market is being flooded with new machines and surgical procedures for mental disorders. Unlike ECT, which is highly effective, these new devices are either ineffective or only marginally helpful. But the companies producing them have rushed them to market, with the complicity of psychiatrists, who are eager to cloak themselves in the medical legitimacy (not to mention the financial rewards) they imply.

A Fork in the Shoulder

In May 2006 the American Psychiatric Association held its 159th annual meeting in Toronto. This was an important moment for the small device company called Cyberonics. One year earlier the FDA had approved a device developed by the company, the vagus nerve stimulator (VNS), as a treatment for depression.[9] Billed as a pacemaker for the brain, the VNS device consists of a silver dollar–sized battery surgically implanted under the skin of the chest. A wire, attached to the battery, is threaded by a surgeon around the vagus nerve in the neck, a nerve which extends into the brain. Once the device is implanted, an external programming box allows a psychiatrist to adjust the settings to release a burst of electricity to the vagus nerve for thirty seconds every five minutes. After this initial setting, the device works autonomously. The patient sees a psychiatrist periodically to fine-tune the settings, and for adjunctive medications and therapy if needed. VNS was approved for patients who are treatment resistant—that is, they continue to suffer even after having tried at least three prior antidepressants or ECT.

But VNS prompted much controversy, because the data in support of the device was weak. Three months before this APA meeting, the *New York Times'* health journalist Gardiner Harris broke the story that although the FDA's expert panel reviewing VNS unanimously voted against approval, their vote was mysteriously overruled by the FDA official in charge of medical devices.[10] In fact, Cyberonics' main study of VNS appeared to show that the treatment was *not* effective for depression. In that study, the company had funded a group of psychiatrists to recruit about two hundred patients with treatment-resistant depression. These patients were randomly assigned to treatment with either VNS or a "sham" version of VNS, in which the device was surgically implanted but was never turned on. This was a double-blind trial, meaning that none of the patients knew whether they were receiving active treatment or sham, nor did the researchers who were rating the depression symptoms. After ten weeks, the response rate for real VNS was 15 percent, while the response rate for sham VNS was 10 percent. This difference, tiny in any case, was not statistically significant, meaning that there was a good chance that the 5 percent separation was a fluke finding. The bottom line was that, according to the usual scientific criteria used to evaluate new treatments, VNS simply didn't work.[11]

After this disappointing study, the patients were allowed to continue in an extension study that lasted for another year. In this study, there was no placebo group, nor was there a double-blind trial. All patients received active VNS, and knew it, as did the symptom raters. From a scientific perspective, this is a huge design flaw, because any improvement could no longer be ascribed to VNS—the influence of other effects, such as hope for a cure and even the positive bias on the part of researchers (who were funded by Cyberonics), would be likely to play a role. At the end of the year, the overall response rate was 27 percent, higher than the 15 percent response rate after ten weeks.[12] But the lack of a placebo group made the 27 percent improvement number impossible to interpret.

When Cyberonics submitted this data, the FDA review team rejected the data as being deficient and asked the company to conduct another placebo-controlled study. But the company said it was "impossible" to conduct such a study (presumably because of the expense), and instead offered data from a different group of depressed patients who had been treated over the course of a year with standard treatments in the community.[13]

At this point, the FDA asked an advisory panel of outside experts to review the new data, and the panel voted 5-2 in favor of approval, a vote in part swayed by emotional testimony from several patients who had been enrolled in the VNS studies. For example, one patient, Charles Donovan, told the panel: "All I can say is that my life is full of genuine happiness and joy. I don't have to fake it anymore. . . . Last Saturday night I attended a small dinner party that 18 months ago I never would have gone to. I am also working on several different projects. This is the most productive I have been in many years."[14]

But one has to take some of this testimony with a grain of salt. Donovan acknowledged that his airfare and lodging were paid for by Cyberonics, and he had made a career out of pro-VNS advocacy, with his own Web site and a book (*Out of the Black Hole: The Patient's Guide to Vagus Nerve Stimulation and Depression*).[15]

Such personal testimonies were likely crucial for approval, because the actual statistics impressed few panel members, even those who voted in favor of approval. For example, Dr. Mary Jensen, a neuroradiologist, explained her yes vote by saying, "Although it would be nice to have randomized controlled data for the efficacy, I believe this is a difficult patient population. . . . And I think [VNS] should at least be available for this group of patients."

This was the sentiment echoed by others: The evidence for efficacy is poor, but the pain of treatment-resistant depression is extreme, so let's go ahead and approve it.

Usually, the members of the FDA's internal review team go along with an advisory committee's recommendation, but in this case they did not. In fact, after once again reviewing the data, they unanimously voted against approval, again asking Cyberonics to conduct a proper controlled study. In response, Cyberonics' fiery CEO, Robert Cummins, went into high gear. In various conference calls and press releases, he insulted FDA's "junior, ill-informed scientists" and suggested that the FDA would now be to blame for the suicides every month of "2,500 people" with treatment-resistant depression. Cummins's passion on this issue is notorious, and may be motivated by the fact that both his mother and grandfather committed suicide.[16]

All eyes were now on the chief of the FDA devices division, Daniel Schultz, who had the ultimate authority to approve a device or not. In a later interview, Schultz said he "agonized" over this decision but ultimately decided to overrule his review team, and the device was approved in February 2005.

This decision was so stunning to the FDA scientists involved that Senator Chuck Grassley of the Senate Finance Committee launched an investigation of the VNS approval process. "In my opinion," wrote one FDA doctor to the committee, "they [Cyberonics] do not have adequate data, and I don't understand how this can move forward." Another reviewer commented, "As an M.D. interested in science, it seems to me that such an approval would be akin to approving an experimental product."

Dr. Peter Lurie of Public Citizen said that the decision was "one of the most questionable regulatory decisions made by the agency in recent memory. As a consequence of the FDA's data-free decision-making," he continued, "hundreds of thousands of patients with severe depression are likely to undergo surgery to implant a device that has not been proved to work."[17]

With so much controversy swirling around VNS, Cyberonics had girded itself for a hard sell at the APA meeting in Toronto, having scheduled a number of lectures by such key opinion leaders as David Dunner and Linda Carpenter and having prepared a large display at the convention center's exhibit hall.[18] As it happened, I learned that Gardiner Harris would be at the conference, and we planned to meet one day in the exhibit hall, an airplane hangar–sized room filled with drug company displays. I promised to give him a guided tour of modern pharmaceutical salesmanship.

Gardiner is a tall man with dark hair cropped neatly at the sides and an affable demeanor belying his status as a crack investigative reporter. He was easy to spot amid the crowd of sports coat–clad psychiatrists swarming through the exhibits and standing in line for freebies.

With a bemused and bewildered smile, he pointed to the Takeda Pharmaceuticals booth next to us. "I have a question. Why is there a woman sleeping in that giant ring?"

There was, indeed, an angelic blond model lying on a bed inside a three-story tall white ring. Her hands were folded together on her stomach, her head was resting on a down-filled pillow, and her eyes were closed. I immediately recognized the image from Takeda's medical journal advertisements for their new sleeping pill, Rozerem. This was an uncanny diorama version. If the company's goal was to attract doctors' attention, they certainly achieved it.

I explained the origin of the display to Gardiner.

"Why the big zero?" he asked.

"That's the Rozerem marketing pitch. It isn't a DEA-controlled substance, unlike most other sleeping pills. In the journals, the ads say: 'Rozerem—ZERO evidence of abuse or dependence.'"

"Now I get it," he said with a chuckle, and we proceeded to wander through the hall, past the booths for Cialis, Lexapro, and Geodon. Smiling and well-scrubbed drug reps were stationed throughout, inviting us to visit.

At the AstraZeneca booth, a rep came up to both of us, hand held out for a shake. He looked at my name tag, flashed me a salesman's smile, and said, "Hello Dr. Carlat." Then he looked at Gardiner's name tag and his smile evaporated.

"Hello there," he said. "I know your name." A bit of the color left his cheeks.

"So," I said, "can we have a look around your exhibit? I have some questions about Seroquel."

"No problem, Dr. Carlat," he said, measuring his words. "We do have someone in the office from media relations if Mr. Harris has any questions."

I asked the rep about some of the data on AstraZeneca's new antipsychotic drug, Seroquel, but as he launched into a canned marketing pitch, my eyes glazed over. As we drifted away, Gardiner said, "I often get that reaction when people from the pharmaceutical industry see my name." I could imagine why. He and his colleagues had written scathing articles about the industry over the years.

Eventually, at the other end of the hall, we came to the Cyberonics booth, where a number of psychiatrists were gathered around displays on VNS. Company reps were pointing at pictures of the device and touting its benefits. Standing next to some of them I noticed the distinguished psychiatrist John Rush, a professor at the University of Texas, who had been the first author of the major Cyberonics-funded research papers that had been argued about during the FDA meetings.

I had recently interviewed him for an issue of *The Carlat Psychiatry Report*,[19] about a separate large antidepressant trial in which Rush had also been a key player, and I brought Gardiner over to meet him.

When I introduced Rush to Gardiner, he did the same *New York Times* double take that I had come to expect by now. I decided to take the opportunity to ask Rush if there was any evidence that the patient improvement reported in the one-year uncontrolled study was due to the VNS device rather than simply due to a placebo response.

Flanked by Cyberonics officials with serious expressions, Rush brought me to a poster outlining the conclusions of the study. Tracing an ascending line on a graph summarizing the results, he commented: "Some have said that this might be a placebo response, but notice how long the improvement lasted, and how it increased over time. Patients with treatment-resistant depression simply don't show this kind of response to placebos."

"But do we have much data about the placebo effect for patients like this?" I asked.

"Not a lot," he admitted. "But I just don't buy that it is the placebo effect."

Rush was referring to the common belief among researchers that although the placebo effect is strong, it is relatively short lived. It is one thing to accept that placebo keeps depression at bay over the course of a six- to ten-week study, but the VNS extension lasted an entire year. To Rush, it seemed unlikely that many of the 27 percent of patients who responded after a year were simply responding to placebo factors.

However, a recent review of long-term antidepressant data found that the placebo response is much longer lasting than had been assumed. In fact, nearly 80 percent of placebo patients who entered long-term extension studies remained perfectly well for up to a year in such studies.[20] The bottom line is that the VNS study results could easily have been explained away as the results of the placebo effect. Rush was exhibiting some wishful thinking in his faith in the data, which was not surprising, especially since the new findings on the durability of the placebo effect were not published until two years after my conversation with him in Toronto.

I thanked Rush for his time, and Gardiner and I walked to the exhibit hall's café for a break. On the way, only a few steps from the Cyberonics exhibit, we passed a small booth where a man was signing books. The contrast between his gray hair and vivacious face struck a chord, and I realized I had seen his photo while researching VNS on the web. This was Charles Donovan, the research subject in the VNS clinical trials who had so effectively testified at the FDA advisory meeting.

On an impulse, I introduced myself to him, admitting to being skeptical of VNS's effects. "The research doesn't seem to show a benefit over placebo," I said.

In response, he spread his arms, palms upraised, smiling radiantly. "Look, if my response is a placebo response, I'll take placebo any day."

It seemed a rather glib statement. If VNS is a placebo, at $25,000 per procedure it would represent the most expensive placebo yet invented. If Donovan truly believed that he had benefited from placebo, it seemed irresponsible of him to be writing books and setting up booths encouraging the world to pay for VNS. But in the interest of collegiality, I kept such thoughts to myself.

Over coffee, Gardiner and I discussed our skepticism about VNS. I told him that I assumed the treatment had been approved under the well-meaning assumption that we needed to be able to offer a very sick group of patients something, even if there was a good chance that it wasn't effective.

Gardiner shook his head, disagreeing. "If the FDA's reasoning for approving VNS was simply that there is no other treatment, they might as well approve sticking a fork into the shoulder of a depressed patient. There's as much evidence for a fork in the shoulder as there is for VNS."

I couldn't argue with his point. And while Cyberonics was initially able to convince plenty of psychiatrists that its "fork in the shoulder" treatment had merit, by 2007 the scientific tide turned against VNS. The *New England Journal of Medicine*, reviewing the same data provided to the FDA, concluded that the "best evidence available to date suggests" that VNS does not work for depression.[21] In May

2007, Medicare finished its own technology review, concluding, like *NEJM*, that VNS was ineffective for depression, and that they would not reimburse patients for the procedure.[22] As is usually the case, private insurance companies followed Medicare's lead, refusing to cover the cost of the treatment, and Cyberonics has essentially given up marketing the device for depression and has returned to its original core business, which is VNS for epilepsy.

The saga of VNS teaches us both about the power of the placebo effect and about the desperation with which psychiatry continues to latch onto unproven treatments. Unfortunately, we have been down this road many times before, having in the past embraced procedures such as insulin coma therapy,[23] transorbital "ice-pick" lobotomies,[24] and even a technique of curing mental illness by removing teeth and internal organs.[25] These bizarre treatments gained popularity because there were no effective alternatives, and because the necessity of placebo-controlled studies was not yet widely appreciated. The same cannot be said now, and I fear the approval of VNS will take its place in history as a blemish on the reputation of both the FDA and American psychiatry.

Transcranial Magnetic Stimulation: A Kinder, Gentler ECT?

The notion that passing magnets over people's heads could make them happier has been around for a very long time, at least since the 1770s. The Viennese physician Franz Anton Mesmer used the technique in front of large eighteenth-century audiences, treating a variety of mental and physical problems by using a combination of iron rods and his own personal "animal magnetism."[26] When treating an individual, he would sit directly in front of him, two sets of knees touching, and would pass his hands over the patient's body to enhance the flow of magnetism. While many endorsed his healing powers, historians now view his treatments as early versions of hypnosis and faith healing. In modern hypnosis, a practitioner uses guided imagery to get patients into a hypnotic, receptive state, and then makes suggestions, such as "When I tell you to wake up, you will feel disgusted every time you see a cigarette." Magnets are no longer part of the procedure.

In the years since, many other claims have been made for the medicinal power of magnets, such as those of Phineas Quimby, the nineteenth-century "magnetic healer" who treated the founder of Christian Science, Mary Baker Eddy.[27] More recently, an entire magnet therapy industry has bloomed, with an array of magnetic rings and bracelets said by their inventors to improve multiple medical problems. So it should not be surprising when a new bold claim about the wonders of magnetism comes up. However, what *is* surprising is when the FDA approves of such a treatment. On October 10, 2008, nearly 250 years after Franz Mesmer wowed his audiences, the FDA did just that, approving of the use of a magnet to treat patients with depression.

The approved device, Neuronetics' NeuroStar Transcranial Magnetic Stimulation machine, looks like a futuristic dentist's chair.[28] Every day for four to six weeks, a patient sits down and a powerful electromagnetic coil is placed on his scalp, radiating a magnetic field into the brain tissue for a half hour. The magnetic field induces a mild electrical current in the neurons, stimulating a specific brain region. Generally, practitioners aim for the left frontal cortex, because some PET scan studies suggest that this area of the brain is underactive in patients with depression.

TMS is billed as a gentler version of ECT, because rather than sending raw electrical current into the brain, TMS uses magnetism to nudge neurons into action. No seizure is induced and no anesthesia is required. There is also no memory loss. Aside from minor scalp itching or pain, the procedure has few side effects, and can be administered by a nurse or a tech in a psychiatrist's office. But does it work?

In the pivotal study of the device—the study that ultimately won it FDA approval—301 depressed patients were randomly assigned to either active TMS or sham TMS; like the study of vagus nerve stimulation, this TMS study was double blind. After four to six weeks of daily TMS treatment (or, in the case of the placebo group, daily sham treatment), both groups got a little bit better. The primary outcome scale used was the MADRS (the Montgomery-Asberg Depression Rating Scale), which is a ten-item questionnaire about the main symptoms of depression. Each depressive symptom, such as sadness, poor concentration, or insomnia, is rated from 0 to 6, with 0 being asymptomatic and 6 being severe. The patients in the TMS studies had an average total score of about 33 before the trial began, which is severely depressed. At the end of the study, the active treatment group improved by 5.8 points, while the placebo group improved by 3.1 points. The difference between the two—2.7 points—is small. Statistically, this difference did not quite reach the level that statisticians consider "significant," which generally implies that a treatment is ineffective.[29]

This was not a particularly impressive result, and an FDA advisory committee initially recommended that TMS be rejected. So why did the FDA approve the device? Did Daniel Schultz overrule the experts again, as he had in 2005 for VNS? No. Instead, Neuronetics did a spectacular reanalysis of their data, with enough slicing and dicing to impress the Iron Chef. They found that if they limited the statistical analysis to only those patients who had failed one prior course of an antidepressant—eliminating about half of the initial number of subjects—then TMS looked pretty effective. In these patients, TMS beat placebo by about 5 points on the MADRS, and this was statistically significant.[30] When the FDA looked at this data in 2008, they decided to approve the device, but only for patients who have tried and failed no more and no less than a single drug trial in the past.

Confused? Basically, what this means is that TMS is effective only for depressed patients who have tried a single antidepressant. The problem with this restriction is that most patients with depression who have not responded to one pill will opt for trying at least one or two other pills before choosing to undergo such a time-intensive treatment as TMS. It is much easier to swallow a pill every morning than it is to have to visit your doctor's office five days a week for six weeks.

Another problem with the treatment is its expense. As is the case for VNS, insurance companies rarely cover TMS treatments. For psychiatrists to recoup the upfront expense of purchasing the NeuroStar TMS device, they must charge patients about $300–$400 per treatment. Given that twenty to thirty daily treatments are needed for improvement in symptoms, the total out-of-pocket cost to a patient is in the range of $10,000. Compared to this, the medication option is dirt cheap. Insurance plans typically cover the cost of psychiatric visits and antidepressants, minus a minimal copay. Therefore, a patient's out-of-pocket cost for standard antidepressant treatment might run about $200 a year, slightly more for psychotherapy. Who would choose to shell out $10,000 instead of $200 for a treatment that is no more effective and is far more time consuming than standard treatment? Only patients who have already tried most antidepressants and who are still depressed. But here's the Catch-22: TMS has not been shown to be effective in such treatment-resistant patients.

One can argue that even if TMS is not very effective, at least it represents a new treatment option, and isn't it better for patients to have more options at their disposal? Such arguments are certainly convenient for the company and for the psychiatrists who might profit from the device. But I don't see it presenting advantages for patients. What I *do* see happening is that clinics offering the treatment are overselling the benefits, evidently in an attempt to recover their upfront investment in the NeuroStar. For example, the Lindner Center for Hope, a clinic near Cincinnati that offers TMS, describes the benefits on its Web site like this:

> Most patients have experienced results by the fourth week of treatment, however each patient is different and some patients may notice benefits over a shorter or longer period of time. In an open-label clinical trial (resembling real world practice) approximately 1 in 2 patients treated with TMS therapy experienced a significant improvement in depression symptoms, and 1 in 3 experienced complete resolution.[31]

The impressive-sounding "open-label clinical trial" refers to an unpublished study conducted by Neuronetics, in which 158 patients were treated with TMS for six weeks and almost half improved.[32] But in this study, there was no placebo group, so the improvement may have been due to the passage of time or other factors unrelated to the magnet's effects. I find it troubling that the Lindner Center would choose not to divulge to prospective patients that in the gold standard placebo-controlled trial, the response rate after six weeks was only 23.9 percent, more than the placebo response rate of 12.3 percent but not at all impressive.

There is nothing inherently wrong with searching for another machine to treat depression. As we've seen, ECT, while effective, has plenty of side effects, and an improved version would be welcome. But when the FDA starts endorsing devices that are ineffective (VNS) or only marginally effective (TMS), there is something wrong with the system, and it needs to be reformed. The FDA's approval criteria should be tightened up, because currently the agency requires far less scientific evidence to approve devices than medications. Companies should not be allowed to statistically manipulate their study results after the fact, as was the case for both VNS and TMS. And most important, we psychiatrists should resist jumping on the device bandwagon because of our misguided professional need to offer a truly "medical" procedure to patients, even when the procedure hardly works.

Peering into the Brain

Patients often ask me if I can give them a brain scan to diagnose what's wrong with them. I wish I could. In mainstream psychiatry, the only accepted use of brain scans is for determining whether a patient might have a brain tumor, a stroke, or some other pathology that could be the cause of a psychiatric symptom. In rare cases, for example, what appears to be psychosis or depression is actually an early symptom of a tumor. Brain scans are excellent at ruling out such neurological problems, so that we can confidently make a psychiatric diagnosis and start appropriate treatment. But these scans cannot actually diagnose depression or schizophrenia, because the responsible brain defects have yet to be discovered.

This is why I was intrigued by a brochure I found in my office mail one day. "Participate in the Imaging Revolution in Psychiatry," it proclaimed. In a "comprehensive 5-day course," psychiatrist Daniel Amen offered to teach psychiatrists how to diagnose conditions by using a type of brain imaging called SPECT scans.[33] Participants would learn how to use brain images to differentiate ADD, depression, dementia, and obsessive compulsive disorder, the flyer said. We could even get our *own* brains scanned at a 20 percent discount. "If you want to know the health of your brain," Amen said in the flyer, "this could be a great opportunity."

Amen owns a chain of clinics that offers comprehensive psychiatric evaluations for $3,300.[34] The price is rather high because, in addition to a series of clinical interviews, it includes two SPECT scans priced at $1,000 each. In several best-selling books, such as *Change Your Brain, Change Your Life* and *Making a Good Brain Great*,[35] Amen has described how he can use scans to diagnose various conditions, such as ADHD, dementia, bipolar disorder, and even PMS (premenstrual symptoms).

But as I read up on Dr. Amen, it was clear that these claims were controversial. He said he has amassed a collection of 42,000 scans over his career, and while he has published some research in medical journals, he has never published the kinds of studies that would scientifically demonstrate the value of the scans. To do this, you would have to compare your diagnosis based on a blind reading of a scan (meaning without having met the patient ahead of time) with the diagnosis of an independent clinical interviewer who had never seen the scan. If there was a high correlation between the two diagnoses, then you would have a convincing new diagnostic test. But Amen has never published such a study.

Critics of Amen are highly skeptical. On the Web site Quackwatch, Dr. Harriet Hall charges that "Dr. Amen claims to be able to choose the best therapy based mainly on scan results, but this claim is supported only by anecdotal evidence and testimonials."[36] Dr. Stephen Hinshaw, chairman of psychology at U.C. Berkeley, likened Amen to a snake oil salesman, saying that "making claims before the evidence is out there does families a lot of harm."[37] The fact that Amen makes money—quite a bit of it, given the success of his clinics—by offering patients SPECT scans is a particular concern. With such an obvious financial interest in the procedure, could he really be expected to be objective in his views?

Eventually, on assignment for an article that was published in *Wired* magazine, I decided to evaluate Amen's procedures myself.[38] I called him in California, telling him that I was writing an article for *Wired* about different brain-scanning techniques, making it clear that I was skeptical. He welcomed my skepticism, seeming to view it as a challenge, and he invited me to his Newport Beach clinic. Thus, in December 2007, I found myself lying down on Amen's scanning table while a camera rotated around my head, halting every thirty seconds or so to take a snapshot. One set of scans, called "concentration scans," was taken just after I concentrated on a computer task, and another, called "resting scans," was taken while I was thinking of nothing in particular.

A SPECT scan is an example of functional neuroimaging, which shows which areas of the brain are most metabolically active at any given time. It is different from a CAT scan and an MRI, which can show only the basic structure of the brain. Using the analogy of a house, structural imaging gives you a static snapshot of the basic layout of your rooms, but functional imaging shows you where people are congregating in real time. SPECT scans (and their more expensive cousins, PET scans) accomplish this through radioactive tracers that concentrate where the brain is active, causing these areas to light up. Thus, these machines provide a direct view of the raw work done by our neurons as we think, feel, and perceive.

After my scan, I met with Dr. Amen, who was a boyish looking man in his fifties sporting a Southern California tan and wearing a black T-shirt, black jeans, and black shoes. This was my third meeting with him in Newport Beach, but our other conversations were about his career and his experiences with other patients. This was the first time we would focus specifically on the meaning of my scans.

I sat on a comfortable couch as he sat at his desk chair, facing me, clipboard in hand. "Today we'll look at both your resting scan and your concentration scan," he said, his expression friendly. "But first, I'd like to go over some of your history."

Amen went through a series of questions I'm accustomed to asking my own patients when I do diagnostic evaluations. He asked me, for example, if I had any history of psychiatric problems. Yes, I suffered a short bout of depression a few years ago, I told him, and had treated myself—successfully—with samples of the antidepressant Celexa. Did I have any medical problems? Nothing significant. Did I have a history of mental illness in my family? I told him about my mother's depression and her eventual suicide.

After another fifteen minutes or so of conversation, he said, "Let's look at your scans." We both walked over to a large round table and he laid out several colorful snapshots of my brain. Red signified areas that were most metabolically active, while blue meant least active. Amen pointed to several views of my brain's surface. "What I see here is that activity in your prefrontal cortex is low at rest, but becomes better when you concentrate, and your thalamus becomes more active too. I think this means that you have a predisposition to depression."

I nodded. Scrutinizing the scans some more, he said, "You need to be busy to be happy. Your brain is cool at rest. You need stuff in your life to feel alive, together, and connected." He paused and looked at me. "I don't know if that fits, but clearly your frontal cortex is low at rest and better when you concentrate."

He looked at another view, this one showing only those brain regions in the top 15 percent of my overall brain activity. "In this scan, you have increased activity in your thalamus, your two basal ganglia, and your cingulate cortex." He picked up a pen and drew a line connecting these four regions. "I call this the 'diamond plus.' It's a pattern of angst, and we see it in people who have had significant trauma in their lives."

"Is this diagnostic of PTSD?" I asked.

"Having the diamond doesn't mean you have PTSD, it means you might have traumatic experiences that you have trouble letting go of."

"Like my mother killing herself?"

"Yes."

"I've never heard of the 'diamond plus' pattern. Is this something you always see in people with trauma?"

"It is not diagnostic of trauma, but it's suggestive. I never say 'This finding equals this,' because in any study there are outliers, people who don't follow the pattern."

I challenged him, pointing out that all of what he had supposedly read in my scans might well have been based on the information he obtained from me during the interview, like my vulnerability to depression or the emotional trauma of my mother's death.

He was unfazed. "Typically I ask clarifying questions, I get your history in my head, then I look at the scans. I don't treat scans, I treat people, and hopefully the scans provide more information."

"But do you have evidence that the scans can provide any additional information beyond the interview?"

Frowning, he said, "I was a psychiatrist for years before I ordered my first scan, and I got tired of making people feel worse. It wears on you. What scans do is give me more info up front before I go about changing somebody's brain. And that's really important for me because I'm often flying blind."

Amen did not answer my question directly, and I was not surprised. I found that typically, when I pressed him on evidence, he would shift to anecdotal stories about patients he had seen and helped, rather than citing studies and statistics. When he did cite evidence, he would allude vaguely to the existence of "thousands of research articles on the topic," but was unable to brandish the crucial kinds of studies that could once and for all prove the validity of his techniques.

I have no doubt that Amen believes that his SPECT scan pictures are valuable, but I believe that they amount to little more than colorful and exorbitantly expensive souvenirs for patients to show their friends. The promise of scans is certainly alluring, but the latest guidelines (from 2006) published by the American Psychiatric Association conclude that "the clinical utility of neuroimaging techniques for planning of individualized treatment has not yet been shown."[39]

Our world is saturated with technology, and it is easy to understand why my colleagues and patients are riveted by the new brain machines. A breathless optimism causes a temporary lockdown on critical abilities, with the result that money and time are wasted on procedures that are about as useful as a fork in the shoulder, and are always more hazardous. Meanwhile, we ignore talk therapy, an unsexy treatment with little commercial potential. But honest and extensive conversation has always been critical for successful healing, in psychiatry and in any other field of medicine. Psychiatrists need to reacquaint themselves with the missing skill of psychotherapy.

Chapter 9

The Missing Skill

In August 2008, the *Archives of General Psychiatry*, which is one of the top two professional journals in the field, published a revealing survey of U.S. psychiatrists.[1]

The researchers found that the percentage of visits to psychiatrists that included psychotherapy dropped from 44 percent in 1996–1997 to 29 percent in 2004–2005. And the percentage of psychiatrists who provided psychotherapy at every patient visit decreased from 19 percent to 11 percent. This decline in therapy was closely correlated with the growth of medication treatment and decreasing insurance reimbursement rates for psychotherapy.

When I saw these figures, I was hardly surprised, as I had watched this trend unfold for the last twenty years. But the media response implied that this was a major new finding. Fox News headlined their coverage "Study: Many Psychiatrists Do Little More Than Write Prescriptions."[2] Reporters scurried around to interview various prominent figures in the field to shed light on the findings. Comments ranged widely.

Some, such as Charles Barber, author of the book *Comfortably Numb: How Psychiatry Is Medicating a Nation*, bemoaned the shift.[3]

"There's almost no marketing for psychotherapy, which has comparable if not better outcomes [than medication]," he said. And Dr. William H. Sledge, the interim chairman of the Yale department of psychiatry, said, "A group of practitioners is losing an important skill. It is like going to war with fewer weapons at your disposal."

On the other hand, Dr. Alan Schatzberg, chairman of the psychiatry department at Stanford University and president-elect of the American Psychiatric Association, was less concerned. He said the trend was not necessarily bad, and could be seen as a natural evolution, part of the progress of science as seen in other fields of medicine. "Years ago, if someone had a herniated disk, they had a very complicated surgical procedure and were in traction for weeks," he said. "Fields change."

From the degree of media interest and the variety of responses, however, a couple of things were clear. First, the public finds it surprising to hear that psychiatrists do not do therapy, and they want to know why. Second, even among psychiatrists, opinions are split about whether the trend is good or bad.

To answer this question, we need to know whether psychotherapy actually works, and whether it works as well as medications. And if it does work, we have to ask why psychiatrists are farming it out. Does this split-treatment approach work? Or should psychiatrists reclaim the skills of psychotherapy?

The public's image of what a therapist does has been shaped by decades of cartoons in *The New Yorker* and elsewhere of a bearded psychiatrist taking notes while the patient lies on a couch. In one memorable version, the psychiatrist has just wordlessly pushed a button on the wall and the couch has catapulted the patient into a hole in the floor.

These cartoons depict the largely outdated version of therapy known as psychoanalysis.[4] As famously introduced by Sigmund Freud, the technique called for a therapist to listen as a patient talked about whatever was on his or her mind, with the therapist making only occasional interjections such as "Uh-huh," "Go on," "Continue that thought," and the infamous, "And how does that make you feel?" Gradually, this technique of free association, it was said, would uncover repressed emotions from the unconscious—rage, fear, sexuality, abject dependency—and as themes emerged, the psychiatrist would jot down notes about them on a pad. The culmination of the process was a pithy interpretation of a patient's dysfunctional approach to life, such as, "You spend your life trying to outperform your father, but when you achieve a real success, you become ashamed and sabotage yourself."

Freud's main contribution was to realize that if a patient was led to explore the important relationship issues in his life within the context of the therapist-patient relationship, that would allow the patient to relive those relationships under the therapist's guidance and to come to powerful realizations about them. In the process, the patient would generally begin feeling and acting in therapy very much the way he acted and felt in his life. As one therapist put it: "The patient eventually brings his whole world into my office. It's not what he tells me that's so important—that's the least accurate information I have. It's how he treats me, and how he feels I'm treating him. I know how he acts with his girlfriend because he acts that way with me some of the time. And I know what goes on with his boss or his kids the same way."[5]

The well-known term for this is "transference," from the fact that the patient transfers habitual ways of perceiving people onto the person of the therapist. The height of the psychoanalyst's art is to be able to perceive transference, and then point it out to the patient in a nonthreatening and productive way. A transference interpretation might be: "Notice how angry you are toward me right now. This is the same kind of anger you have toward your boss, and the same anger you had toward your father when he failed to respond to your needs. Perhaps there are better ways to get your needs met?"

Over the decades, psychoanalysis has morphed into a modern version called psychodynamic therapy.[6] Now, therapist and patient both sit in chairs and face one another. The therapist is more active, and therapy moves along more quickly. Insights can be achieved in months instead of years. In the HBO show *In Treatment*, the therapist Paul Weston, played by Gabriel Byrne, practices the new psychodynamic therapy, constantly confronting patients with their behavior.[7] If they change the subject to avoid a topic, he tells them what they are doing; if a woman is flirting with him, he points out the behavior and wonders why it is happening, and what the behavior says about the patient's personality. While Dr. Weston's sessions are far more dramatic than real psychotherapy, they are essentially accurate depictions of the best of modern psychodynamic therapy.

Recently, another type of therapy has emerged and is threatening to supplant psychodynamic therapy as the preferred technique. It has become so popular that *Forbes* magazine devoted its April 2007 cover article to it, proclaiming: "Dump the couch! And ditch the Zoloft. A new therapy revolution is here."[8]

This "revolution" is cognitive behavioral therapy (CBT), a technique devised by a disenchanted psychoanalyst named Aaron Beck. Beck became impatient with the glacial pace of progress in psychoanalysis, and decided that a more efficient way to get patients to feel better is to teach them how to *think* better. Instead of asking "How does that make you feel," he began asking patients "How does that make you think?" He found that depression and anxiety are often triggered by irrational thoughts and ideas. If patients could identify their distorted thoughts and question them, they could presumably change the negative emotions the thoughts had triggered.

CBT has been studied by comparison with medications and has been found to be equally effective for depression and anxiety disorders. In some cases, it is more effective, especially for preventing relapses over the long term.[9] One of its most widely acknowledged uses is in treating panic disorder, and I've applied it for that problem myself.

In October 2007, my wife and I boarded a commuter plane in Washington, D.C., bound for Boston. The plane had only twenty rows of seats, and when the flight crew closed the hatch, the air became hot and stuffy. Washington was in the midst of a heat wave, and the airplane's weak air conditioning was fighting a losing battle with a tropical 90 degrees on the tarmac.

I suddenly felt the need to take deeper breaths and then I was seized with the thought that I needed to leave. I found myself thinking, "If I don't get off this plane right now, I'm going to suffocate." At that moment, the captain announced that the flight was delayed by a half hour. Now I really felt trapped, and I began taking deeper breaths. My chest felt tight, my pulse quickened, and as I hyperventilated, I felt lightheaded. I knew I was having a panic attack.

I treat patients with panic disorder all the time, but the treatment I knew best involved SSRIs like Zoloft or benzodiazepines like Xanax, and I had no Xanax. In residency, I had taken seminars in cognitive behavior therapy, but it had been many years since I had used it for patients. Sitting there, hyperventilating, claustrophobic, heart pounding, I racked my brain, trying to remember the CBT techniques for calming myself down.

I knew I had to identify my inaccurate thoughts. That was easy enough. I realized that I could not actually be about to suffocate. So I said to myself, "Be rational. You're not suffocating. You are having a panic attack." I then lectured myself, "You know what a panic attack is. It's an irrational fear reaction. You are hyperventilating because of fear, not because of lack of oxygen."

By counting my inhalations and exhalations I began to regularize my breathing. I also reminded myself that panic attacks have a beginning, middle, and an end. They inevitably subside. Another technique then came to mind: distraction. I picked up the inflight magazine, forcing my neurons to focus on an article about ecotourism in Costa Rica. Gradually, very gradually, I began to feel better.

After returning home, this powerful experience forced me to rethink how I was practicing my craft. I had known for many years that new psychotherapy techniques were being shown to be as effective as medications in some disorders, and at times even *more* effective. Why was I not offering these techniques to my patients? Had I undergone eight long years of medical and psychiatric training just to be a pill pusher?

One reason so few psychiatrists spend significant time doing therapy is that they will earn less by doing so. For example, for years I typically saw three patients per hour, and was reimbursed about $60 per visit, depending on the insurance plan. This worked out to about $180 an hour, although when you factor in canceled or missed appointments, office rent, a billing service, and so on, my take-home was closer to about $130 an hour.

If I did therapy, I could see one patient in that hour, and insurance companies reimbursed anywhere from $80 to $100 for that visit. After expenses, this came down to around $70/hour. The bottom line is if I did therapy exclusively, I would have to take a 40–50 percent pay cut. Most psychiatrists, like me, choose a psychopharmacology practice.

Nonetheless, many psychiatrists actually want to do more therapy, and there is a long-standing battle between psychiatrists and managed care companies over their reimbursement policies. Managed care companies discourage us from doing psychotherapy, arguing that it is more cost effective for psychiatrists to do 15-minute medication visits every 3 months, and to hire a lower paid non-M.D. for more frequent therapy visits. Not enough research has been done to evaluate this claim, but the few studies that have been published suggest that integrated treatment actually saves money. For example, Mantosh Dewan, the chairman of psychiatry at SUNY Syracuse, found that when psychiatrists do both medication and psychotherapy, the overall amount of money paid out by insurance companies is actually less than when the treatment is split between psychiatrists and therapists.[10] When patients see only one provider, they require fewer visits overall.

Of course psychiatrists who want to do therapy are free to do as much as they want; that just depends on how much less money they are willing to make. One of my colleagues, a psychiatrist based in rural Vermont named Alice Silverman, decided early in her career that she wanted to combine therapy and psychopharmacology. In order to be able to afford medical school, she signed up for a program in which the National Health Service Corps funded her training. In return, she agreed to work in an underserved area for at least three years. She set up shop in St. Johnsbury, Vermont, and never left.

Silverman worked for a mental health center initially, seeing patients for thirty-minute visits—which is long for a psychiatric visit, but still not long enough for her to accomplish the work she longed to do. "I saw that many of my patients lived in poverty-stricken, oppressive life circumstances," she recalls, "and I decided that I wasn't simply going to treat them by medicating them."

In her private practice she schedules all of her patients for fifty-minute sessions in which she integrates psychotherapy and psychopharmacology.

"If patients have severe symptoms, I don't hesitate to medicate," she told me. "But most of the people I see have misery and unhappiness, rather than major depression. They are miserable because of problems in relationships or difficulties coping with their life's circumstances. Therapy can be very helpful for them."

"Aren't you taking a financial hit?" I asked. She nodded. "I made about $82,000 in salary last year." That was about half what a full-time psychiatrist in private practice typically makes.

"How does it feel giving up that extra $80,000 a year?"

"We do perfectly fine financially," she said. (She is married to a social worker.) "I love my work. I could be doing brief medication visits, but there's a confidence and a trust that is very hard to develop with fifteen-minute visits. I have a deep connection with my patients, and that's very powerful."

I asked her to give me an example of how her integrated treatment worked, and she told me about a patient she had just seen that morning, a man in his fifties who recently had cancer surgery. His wife had referred him because of his anxiety. "He woke up every morning with anxiety so severe that he was gagging," Alice recounted. "He didn't want to move, and he began having dark, suicidal thoughts."

"Sounds like he had an agitated depression," I said. "What did you do?"

"I started him on an SSRI initially. But he had side effects. He was already on Klonopin when I saw him, but if anything, he was using too much of it. He couldn't socialize without it. Part of his anxiety was actually caused by his dependence on that drug. So we agreed to gradually taper it."

"How did you manage that?" I asked. Klonopin, a highly addictive benzodiazepine, is notoriously hard to discontinue.

"I used CBT [cognitive behavioral therapy]."

"And were you fairly proficient in CBT?" I asked.

"Yes, because I made a concerted effort to train myself in it. I learned CBT because I had a lot of socially anxious patients who weren't getting better with medications. I went to conferences and workshops."

I myself had received a fair amount of CBT training at Mass General, where I had taken a workshop taught by another psychiatrist, Steve McDermott. But once I got busy with my private practice, I found, for various reasons, that I wasn't using the technique. I spent so much of my time with patients talking about medications and their side effects that I lost my CBT skills by attrition.

Alice Silverman put her finger on the crux of the problem beautifully when she said to me, "Why would you choose psychiatry just to give people psychotropic medication? I'm assuming if you go into psychiatry you're really interested in the mind."

When my father did his residency at San Francisco's Langley Porter Psychiatric Institute in the 1950s, he learned therapy well, because, with few medications available, therapy was the main treatment psychiatrists could offer their patients. Psychiatric residencies focused on therapy, and many residents extended their training further by enrolling in postgraduate psychoanalytic institutes. When modern medications came on the scene, my father adapted by incorporating them into his therapy practice, as did many of his colleagues. I call this the "lost" generation of psychiatrists, those currently approaching retirement age, who were skilled at offering the full package of effective psychiatric treatments to patients.

I asked him how he managed to do as much therapy as his did and still make a good income. According to surveys, roughly one-third of all U.S. psychiatrists no longer accept managed care insurance payments, requiring that patients pay their fees out of pocket.[11] Patients can then try to recoup some of the costs directly from their insurance companies, which is always a challenging task. But my father, like me, continues to accept almost all health insurance plans.

It turns out that he can afford to do therapy by creative scheduling. Rather than scheduling patients within standard one-hour blocks, he chooses 45-minute blocks, in which he schedules either two medication visits or one therapy visit. Thus, he spends from 20 to 25 minutes with his medication patients, somewhat longer than the standard 15-minute med-check visits. He believes those extra few minutes make a difference, allowing him to do a better assessment of symptoms. And while 45 minutes may not sound like a very long therapy session, most insurance companies consider a standard therapy visit to be 45 to 50 minutes (hence, the so-called 50-minute hour). Limiting therapy visits to 45 minutes has the effect of allowing him to fit in more medication visits over the course of a day. For him, this was a perfect compromise between his desire to spend enough time with patients to truly help them, and his need for a decent income.

Inspired by him, I began experimenting with a similar type of schedule in my practice. In the past, my 20-minute medication appointments consisted of getting specific bullets of information—"Have you had any medication side effects? How are your symptoms? Any other concerns? Do you need refills?" But during my longer sessions (which are now 20 to 25 minutes for medication visits, and 45 minutes for therapy visits), I have the time to ask about my patients' lives. "How is your relationship with your husband? Has anything been bugging you about your job? What have you been doing for fun?"

As I began this new style of practicing, the first thing that struck me is that I had barely known many of my patients. I had exuberantly documented their moods, sleep habits, energy levels, and whether they had suicidal thoughts, but I didn't know what made them tick as people. For example, I had treated June, a health care administrator in her forties, for depression and bulimia for many years, focusing on a complicated combination of medications such as Effexor, Provigil, amitriptyline, and Xanax. During one visit, she told me her depression had returned. Rather than simply asking about symptoms and making a medication adjustment, I took the time to ask her what was going on in her life. I found out that her boss had recently given her an impossible assignment to complete, and had berated her when the results were not to his liking. It seemed clear to me that her depression was partly triggered by the fact that she blamed herself for her boss's poor communication skills and managerial lapses.

"Why are you blaming yourself?" I asked her.

It turned out that self-blaming had become an automatic habit of June's thinking. When something went wrong, she assumed it was her fault.

I encouraged her to take a step back and question that assumption each time it popped into her mind. Over the next few visits, she improved significantly—relating better to her boss, able to take his criticism with a grain of salt, and feeling more confident.

But, as is true in most patients, the plot thickened. While my simple therapeutic suggestions were helpful, as June and I continued to explore her work issues in detail, she admitted that she often lacked focus on the job. Knowing that poor concentration can be a symptom of depression, I asked if she associated her distractibility with periods of sadness. But she said there was no such correlation with her moods.

I wondered if she might have an adult version of attention deficit hyperactivity disorder (known as ADHD). Indeed, carefully reviewing her years in school, it was clear that she had always been flighty and easily distracted, but had overcome this problem by working extra hard and had managed to achieve good grades. Even now, her job performance was consistently rated as excellent, but the extra work this entailed sapped her energy.

I decided to prescribe her a version of Ritalin, the standard treatment for ADHD. The next month, she felt that this medication had turned her life around. Not only did she feel more focused and productive at work, but she was more apt to get things done at home, which in turn enhanced her mood, indirectly improving her depression.

The kind of psychotherapy I provided June did not fit the traditional model of weekly hour-long sessions probing the roots of her personality traits and drawing connections with her family of origin. Instead, it was a version of supportive therapy that I now try to weave into the fabric of all my sessions with patients, whether they are seeing me primarily for medications or for therapy. In

June's case, spending a bit more time understanding her accomplished two things.

Therapeutically, it allowed me to address the psychological aspects of her depression, but it also improved the medication part of her treatment, because the extra information I gleaned led to a successful trial of Ritalin.

Increasingly, it seems to me that the very term "psychopharmacologist" may be doing more harm than good to the field of psychiatry. The American Society of Clinical Psychopharmacology (ASCP) defines psychopharmacology on its Web site as "the study of the use of medications in treating mental disorders."[12] But in a recent article, three Harvard psychiatrists (two of them, ironically, from Mass General) have pointed out that no other medical specialty has carved out a separate subspecialty called "pharmacology." Good doctoring, they remind us, involves perfecting all the skills relevant to healing and deploying them when needed.[13] This is a far cry from organizing one's practice into fifteen-minute "med checks."

To be fair, most psychopharmacologists do, in fact, provide therapy to most of their patients, though they may not consciously label it as such.

The simple act of confession is a kind of "accidental" therapy practiced by all psychiatrists. This is a technique we share with the clergy. Recently, for example, a married woman came in for an initial appointment and, with a sense of shame and embarrassment, told me about a coworker with whom she had had an affair. The man had just announced that he wanted their relationship to end. Though devastated, she could not share the source of her pain with her husband, and she was suffering from depression. At the end of our appointment, she said, "You know, I feel so much better just having told you about this." She later canceled her next appointment, telling me she felt so improved after the evaluation that she no longer needed treatment.

Even providing patients with a diagnosis, which psychiatrists typically do at the end of the first visit, is a form of therapy. Part of what makes mental illness so painful is its terrible mystery. Patients in the midst of a crisis feel that they are spinning out of control, do not know what they are experiencing, and wonder if they will ever feel normal again. Providing them with an explanation goes a long way toward a cure. "Part of the service we provide to people is to offer them a formal diagnosis," said Michael Posternak, a colleague who sees patients in his private practice. "A new patient came in the other day, I did my usual evaluation, and then I gave her my formal diagnostic summary—major depression, social anxiety, and borderline personality disorder. After discussing these syndromes in detail, she broke down in tears, saying that it all made sense now."

Of course these forms of therapy are quite limited in their effect, especially for the more complex problems. Quite a few psychiatrists do offer an amount of actual talk therapy, though the time given to it is much shorter than in classic therapy. Posternak, for example, who sees patients for fifteen-minute appointments, told me, "If you tape-recorded these sessions, the first twelve minutes or so cover psychological issues, the last three minutes are about medications."

I do the same thing during my twenty-minute appointments. Another patient, Ellen, was going through a difficult time because of impending heart surgery. I had her on Lexapro for depression and anxiety, and Ambien for insomnia. During one recent twenty-five minute visit, she told me the meds were helping, but that she felt very bad about a recent conversation with her husband. "He said that I was really out of shape and that I looked awful." The comment had festered. She felt bad about the comment, but she felt even worse about the fact that her husband, whom she loved so dearly, had said it. Though she wanted to talk to him about it, she feared making the situation worse. I suggested we role-play a conversation in which she would tell him how hurt she had felt, while at the same time pointing out that there was a good reason she was out of shape, namely, that she had a bad heart and was chronically fatigued. She left the session feeling encouraged.

My simple little intervention might be called therapy/lite. If true psychotherapy is like marshaling an army to combat lifelong patterns of negative behavior, the mini-therapy of modern psychiatrists is like launching a single missile for a surgical strike. It accomplishes a limited objective, but it's not enough to get the job done.

In my opinion, the greatest disservice psychiatrists do is to encourage patients to open themselves up and then to slam the door shut when they are at their most vulnerable. This often happens during the first session, ostensibly devoted to generating a DSM diagnosis. After we've asked our series of questions to rule in or rule out symptoms, we typically probe no further into patients' answers, which can be indicating very serious problems. A common question in evaluating depression is "Are you still able to enjoy things that you used to enjoy?" A "no" means that the patient has the symptom of anhedonia. Recently, I asked this question and the patient, a forty-eight-year-old electrician, was thrown for a loop. "What did I used to enjoy?" he repeated after I asked. "I haven't thought about that," he said. "I used to read more. I used to play poker with the guys. I don't do any of those things anymore." He wanted to dwell on this topic, finding it fascinating. But I needed to move on in order to be able to complete the interview before my next patient sounded the chime. If he wanted to follow up on the topic of how his life had changed over the years, he would have to call a therapist to whom I would refer him. At least I would give him a referral.

Good therapists often say that it is vital to "strike while the iron is hot." But modern psychiatry is set up to turn the heat up and then plunge the iron into ice-cold water.

Fragmented Care versus Integrated Care

The strange division of labor between prescribers and therapists has been charitably called the "split treatment" model of care, but a more accurate term is "fragmented care."

A key problem with "split" treatment is that it often amounts to half treatment, because patients dislike having to see a second provider. It is not easy, after all, to pour out your soul to a stranger, and patients sometimes balk at my suggestion that they do it all over again to another stranger. There are also logistical barriers to overcome. Our complicated managed care insurance system means that each company has its own panel of providers, and the therapists I recommend may not be on that panel. Or, patient and therapist may not be able to coordinate their schedules. Or, the patient may not like the way the therapist sounds on the phone. It is easy to get spooked by someone who will be expecting you to divulge your deepest secrets.

Another problem is that once a patient is hooked up with a therapist, I have no way of knowing whether the therapist is skillful, nor do I know what issues they are working on. Ideally, I would be able coordinate care with the therapist by chatting or e-mailing frequently, but with my caseload of hundreds of patients, this is impossible. A therapist may even work at cross-purposes with what I am trying to accomplish.

For example, Shirley was a woman with depression and multiple personality disorder who had been abused badly as a child, including episodes of having been locked in a closet for days at a time. She saw a therapist who had her repetitively relive these experiences, with the goal of eventually depriving the memories of their traumatic power. Theoretically, this is a solid therapeutic strategy, and research has proven its effectiveness in post-traumatic stress disorder. However, it was not working for Shirley, who told me she was having intense desires to cut herself. I would increase her medication in order to help her manage the impulses, but with limited success. After a couple of weeks of trading voice messages, I discussed my concerns with her therapist, who agreed it was time to tone down the intensity of the therapy.

Of course this problem works both ways. Sometimes *I* am the one who is missing something important. In one case, I found out that a patient had been violent to his wife only after finding out he had been arrested. The patient's therapist had known more about his history of past violence, information that I had not learned during our short sessions. In another case, I found out that one of my patients, an elderly woman, had been drinking heavily every night to get to sleep, on top of the sleeping pills I prescribed. This had been going on for many months before the therapist called me to make sure I was aware of it. At the next session, I brought this up and together we devised an outpatient detox plan. It was sheer luck that no serious harm had been done, because the combination of alcohol and sleeping pills is known to sometimes cause patients to stop breathing.

Our system of fragmented care is a dangerous game. The fact is that medication treatment and therapy treatment interact with one another. The more I know about my patient's psychology, the better my medication decisions will be.

Ultimately, there is no inherent reason for psychiatrists to be considered "biological" practitioners and psychologists and social workers to be called "psychological" practitioners. Scott Waterman, a psychiatrist and dean of students at the University of Vermont Medical School, has written about this false dualism permeating psychiatric thought, which he considers a throwback to Descartes's seventeenth-century belief that mind and body are distinct entities. Waterman has studied the philosophy of psychiatry and we discussed some of his ideas recently.

"If you ask most psychiatrists if they think there was a difference between mental and physical," he began, "they would say 'No, we realize that all thoughts and moods are related to some chemical changes in the brain.' But if you were a fly on the wall you would hear them talk to patients about how, for example, some aspects of their depression (such as insomnia) are 'biological,' while other aspects (such as their self-deprecating thoughts) are 'psychological.' Then, they might propose a biological treatment for the former and psychological treatment for the latter. The problem, though, is that the categories 'biological' and 'psychological' do not refer to different underlying processes, but instead refer to different perspectives on, or ways of talking about, the same processes."

As an oft-cited example of this idea, Waterman described studies on obsessive compulsive disorder (OCD) in which researchers used PET scans to track changes in brain metabolism in OCD patients who had been randomly assigned to receive either medication or cognitive behavioral therapy.[14] Among those patients whose symptoms (for example, excessive hand washing and checking) improved with treatments, subsequent PET scans found precisely the same brain metabolism changes—namely, a reduction in the hyperactivity of a certain neural circuit—regardless of whether the treatment was pharmacological or behavioral. As much as it may be convenient and intuitive for us to use the language of dualism, in fact psychopharmacologists and psychotherapists are both treating the same thing—what we might call the mind/brain.

As I talked to Waterman about these concepts, I was reminded of a basic disagreement between therapists and psychopharmacologists that still comes up occasionally. Psychiatrists sometimes say that therapy "ignores" the underlying biological problem, while therapists often counter that psychiatric medications simply put a Band-Aid on symptoms without addressing the deeper psychological issues. The fact is, however, that these are simply two different ways of approaching the same underlying problems, and there is no reason to believe that one is superior to the other.

While this does not imply that a single practitioner should be in charge of both the medications and the psychotherapy, I believe that we would do a better job with our patients if we took an integrated approach. Actually accomplishing this on a large scale will be a challenge. The issues are complex and the possible solutions are many, as we will next explore.

Chapter 10

Solutions

In order to fix the many problems explored in this book, I believe the profession must develop a vision of the ideal psychiatrist. After hearing a patient pour out his or her soul, this is what I believe the ideal psychiatrist should be able to say in response:

"I've listened to you carefully, and I believe I understand exactly what you have been going through. I've seen many people who have faced similar challenges, and I have expertise in all the major techniques for treating psychological problems. I understand how to match psychiatric medications to your symptoms, but I also understand their limitations. I do not accept any money or other incentives from the pharmaceutical industry, because I want to do what is best for you and not what is best for a drug company. I also have much more to offer you than a series of medications trials. I have learned the most effective techniques of psychotherapy, and I will deploy these methods when they are needed. My philosophy is that each patient is unique in their needs, and I will find just the right mix of therapy and medication to help you to move beyond the difficulties that seem so overwhelming."

Sadly, the integrative practitioner who could honestly say these things is rare. Why should this be? This chapter is about understanding what has prevented our medical community and our society from producing the best mental health practitioners on earth—and about how to start creating ideal psychiatrists now.

The Turf Wars

On February 18, 2005, in Baton Rouge, Louisiana, Dr. John Bolter wrote out a prescription for a patient and thereby made a kind of history. "She was an older woman who had chronic pain problems," he recalled. "She had been depressed, was not sleeping well, and had not been eating. I prescribed her Remeron Sol-tabs because she said she hated swallowing pills."[1]

"How did she do on the medication?" I asked.

"She did well. I chose it because of Remeron's side effects of sedation and increased appetite, and in fact she started eating again and sleeping well."

This made sense. It was one of those circumstances when you can make a rational medication decision based on the side-effect profile. I, too, have found Remeron helpful for elderly patients with insomnia and weight loss due to depression.

So why did this make history? Because Bolter is no psychiatrist, and in fact has no medical degree at all. He is a PhD psychologist. John Bolter was the first psychologist in U.S. history to prescribe a medication under a state law granting psychologists limited prescriptive privileges.

This issue brings the blood of psychiatrists to a boil like none other. Soon after Louisiana allowed psychologists like Bolter to prescribe a small number of psychiatric drugs, then-APA president Michelle Riba called such laws "assaults on safe patient care" and said that "terrible things are going to happen [to patients] as a result of this." Her article outlining psychiatry's response was titled "APA

Armed and Ready to Fight Psychologist-Prescribing Bills."[2] At a recent meeting I attended in Massachusetts, a colleague, generally as mellow as a summer breeze, said the idea of psychologists prescribing was an "abomination." I had to glance at him twice to make sure the words had actually come from his mouth. This was really tribal warfare.

The idea of psychologists prescribing medications may sound alarming at first, because we are accustomed to the idea that only physicians should have the power to prescribe. However, doctors' hegemony over the prescription pad has been eroding at an accelerating rate over the past few decades. This trend began in the 1960s, when a critical shortage of doctors led to the emergence of nurse practitioners (NPs) and physician's assistants (PAs), both of whom can write prescriptions. By 1990 there were twenty-eight thousand NPs in the United States, and the demand for these "physician-extenders" has kept growing—by the year 2000 the total number of NPs had mushroomed to seventy-seven thousand.[3]

One of the educational tracks for NPs is a psychiatric track. Graduates are called "psychiatric clinical nurse specialists," and they can do almost everything psychiatrists can do. They can hang a shingle and start a private practice, they can prescribe without direct physician supervision, and they can bill insurance companies for their services. When these psychiatric NPs first came on the scene in the early 1990s, "psychiatrists were aghast," according to one NP I interviewed, who asked to remain anonymous.

"The psychiatrists were threatened by us," she said. "At the drug company–funded dinner lectures, the psychiatrists would sit on one side of the room, and we would sit on the other." Eventually, this tense relationship softened considerably, presumably because it turned out that there was plenty of business to go around. Furthermore, psychiatrists eventually found that NPs could actually become a financial boon for them in various ways. Some hire NPs to see excess patients in their practices, taking a percentage of their insurance reimbursement fees. Others charge up to $300/hour to supervise the NPs, which can amount to a lucrative source of income in some communities.

Meanwhile, dozens of studies of NPs have found that they provide care competently and safely—despite the fact that they receive less than a third of the medical training of physicians. It turns out that you *can* safely prescribe without going to medical school, as long as you get the proper training in a certified educational program. Psychiatric clinical nurse specialists are now an accepted and uncontroversial part of the medical community.

Now the turf wars are being fought between psychiatrists and psychologists. As was the case for nurse practitioners, the concept of giving psychologists prescribing privileges was hatched because of a shortage of physicians.

In 1991, the Department of Defense, realizing that they were unable to retain enough psychiatrists in the military to meet the clinical demand, developed an experimental program to teach psychologists how to prescribe medications. The two-year training began with a year of classroom courses in physiology and pharmacology—similar to courses medical students take over their first two years, but whittled down to those of most relevance to psychiatry. The second year was on-the-job training with supervision, essentially an abbreviated version of a psychiatric residency. Over the seven-year life-span of the program, a total of ten psychologists were graduated, eventually working as prescribers of a limited formulary of psychiatric medications.

How did these pioneers do? In 1998, the program was evaluated by the American College of Neuropharmacology, which is a group of hard-nosed biologically oriented psychiatrists involved in research and teaching.[4] This panel visited the clinical settings where the psychologists practiced, interviewing the trainees, their supervising physicians, and other staff involved. In their final eighty-six-page report, the panel concluded that the program was an unqualified success. According to their report, all ten graduates "performed with excellence wherever they were placed," and there were no reports of medication errors or bad patient outcomes.[5]

Surprisingly, these psychiatrists felt that only two years of training was sufficient, stating in their executive summary that "it seems clear to the Evaluation Panel that a 2-year program—one year didactic, one year clinical practicum that includes at least a 6-month inpatient rotation—can transform licensed clinical psychologists into prescribing psychologists who can function effectively and safely in the military setting. . . ." To be sure, the trainees' medical knowledge was weaker than psychiatrists'—something that was also mentioned in the report. But the psychologists were aware of their limitations and made appropriate referrals to primary care doctors when necessary. On the other hand, in one case the panel noted that a graduate was *more* knowledgeable about psychiatric medications than his psychiatrist supervisor.

Ultimately, this training program was discontinued because the General Accounting Office determined that the military already had enough psychiatrists and that training psychologists to prescribe was an unnecessary expense.[6] But in civilian society, there continues to be a severe shortage of psychiatrists[7] (especially outside of big cities) and the American Psychological Association, emboldened by the DoD demonstration project, created a series of civilian psychology training programs loosely modeled on the military's curriculum. Lobbyists for the group have fanned out to state legislatures, arguing that psychologists should be given limited prescription privileges. Thus far, they have had most success in largely rural states where psychiatrists are rare. New Mexico authorized a psychology prescribing law in 2001, Louisiana in 2004, and Oregon is likely to pass such a law sometime in 2010 or 2011.

In both New Mexico and Louisiana, the experience with prescribing psychologists has been similar to the army's program. According to John Bolter, there are currently fifty psychologists licensed to prescribe in Louisiana, and about ten are graduating from the psychopharmacology master's program per year. Thus far there have been no adverse health outcomes or patient complaints related to these practitioners. And while psychiatrists in the state are unhappy about having lost the legislative battle, apparently they are accommodating to the changed landscape, realizing that they are not losing any business. "As you know, there is plenty of this kind of work to go around," said Bolter, who works in a practice specializing in neurological illnesses.

A Profession Under Siege

What do these developments mean for psychiatry as a profession?

I spoke about this to Richard Cooper, a physician and professor of medicine at the University of Pennsylvania. Cooper is considered the guru of the study of medical professions, having presciently predicted in the 1980s that a major shortage of physicians was looming in most specialties. I got Dr. Cooper on the phone one day and I asked him about his thoughts on the future of psychiatry.

Of all specialties, Cooper finds psychiatry the hardest to predict. "This is because the margins between what psychiatrists do and what others in the mental health professions do is much less clear than in other specialties," said Cooper. He notes that, historically, medical specialties develop control over their profession by developing a specialized body of knowledge that defines their turf, guarding against interlopers from other fields.

But psychiatry is an exception to this process, Cooper has written. "Rather than seizing new problems that emerge from technological progress or conceptual growth, it has expanded its scope of interest by medicalizing what are often referred to as 'problems of living.'"[8] Cooper is not arguing that problems such as ADHD or social anxiety are not real—like me, he has no doubt that many who receive these diagnoses have true psychiatric illness. He is arguing that while other specialties such as cardiology, surgery, or radiology have developed by creating new knowledge and new procedures, psychiatry has grown by bringing more existing disorders into its sphere of influence. This is a tough way to define a profession, because each time you try to drag one of these diagnoses into your profession, you are essentially taking it away from some other specialty that has already laid claim to it. For example, in the realm of ADHD, therapists and pediatricians are already centrally involved in treating such children. In the realm of depression, a whole slew of professionals can lay claim to effective treatment—psychologists, social workers, nurses, priests, and so on.

A profession that defines itself in this way becomes porous; its boundaries become fuzzy. It leaves itself highly vulnerable to marauders from other fields—like, for example, nurses and psychologists.

The solution, of course, is not to build the walls higher, nor is it to station guards with powerful weaponry on the ramparts. This is the strategy that psychiatry is now using—deploying lobbyists to battle everyone from psychologists to insurance companies. The real solution is to make the profession more impressive and scientific. If you develop a professional knowledge base that is truly unique, specialized, and useful to the public, the pretenders to the inner sanctum will be defrocked by their obvious lack of that knowledge.

One obvious solution is to put more funds into neurobiological research, but we may be decades away from reaping the fruits of that research, and meanwhile we have a profession that is being deconstructed before its eyes.

What is to be done?

A Menu of Solutions

The essential problem with psychiatry is that it is hyper-focused on psychopharmacology at the expense of other effective techniques. Any solution must lead to mental health practitioners who can expertly decide what the best treatment is for a particular patient, and then implement that treatment.

Does this mean that all psychiatrists should take a full hour for each patient, always doing both psychotherapy and medication prescribing? Not at all. For some patients, a fifteen-minute check-in and a prescription is perfectly adequate.

Some months ago, a historic drawbridge spanning the Merrimac River was damaged when a barge smashed into a part of it. Since then it has been closed, and my patients from across the river must drive several miles out of their way to find an alternative route to my office in Newburyport. They are often late. Marianne, for example, is a woman with bipolar disorder who recently arrived twenty minutes late for her twenty-minute time slot. Out of breath, she plopped herself down and apologized, then said, "Anyway, I'm fine, I just need my meds." Having known Marianne now for ten years, I could tell immediately that she was, in fact, feeling good, thinking clearly, functional, and engaging with life normally. She was neither manic nor depressed. I wrote prescriptions for her three medications and she was out of the office in five minutes.

Other times, the opposite situation occurs. A patient came in for a twenty-minute follow-up appointment. She said the Ativan I had just prescribed was not quite working for her anxiety. I asked a few questions, and decided to prescribe her Klonopin because it is more long-acting. I wrote the prescription as I heard my next patient entering the waiting room, and as I handed it to her, I saw that she was crying. "What's going on?" I asked. It turned out that a lot was going on, much more than I had imagined. She hated her job and she hated her life. She felt stuck. Today, she needed more than twenty minutes of psychopharmacology talk—and I gave her that extra time, figuring that I would be able to make it up later in the day by budgeting less time for a patient who was stable.

Since I reengineered my schedule, I have more flexibility to take the time I need for a particular patient. I still have plenty of patients whom I see primarily for medication and who see a social worker or psychologist for therapy. Sometimes split treatment works fine, but I am no longer able to tolerate having a practice consisting entirely of psychopharmacology clients. On the other hand, if I insisted on taking over the psychotherapy for all of my patients, I would not have time to see them all, and would have to refer many of them to other treaters—something I'd prefer not to do, both because of the hassle involved and because I am attached to patients I have come to know and like.

My logistical challenges illustrate how hard it is for psychiatrists to introduce therapy into their practices after they have been at it for a couple of decades. This is why we need creativity if we want to devise the ideal mental health system.

Here are some of our options.

1. Continue the status quo.

We can choose to leave the system as is, and simply encourage psychiatrists to think more broadly about what they do. This process has already begun. For example, in 2001, the ACGME (Accreditation Council for Graduate Medical Education) instituted a requirement that all psychiatry residencies add cognitive behavioral therapy to the curricula.[9] In a later survey published in 2006, it was reported that 90 percent of residencies had complied with the requirement.[10]

Unfortunately, requiring psychotherapy training in a psychiatry residency hardly guarantees that the graduates will actually do therapy when they graduate. Psychiatric residencies have long been required to offer training in various forms of therapy. The American Board of Psychiatry and Neurology, which writes the exams for licensure, publishes a list of "core competencies" required of psychiatrists.[11] We are expected to have the ability to "conduct a range of individual, group, and family therapies using standard, accepted models, and to integrate these psychotherapies in multi-modal treatment, including biological and sociocultural interventions." These requirements have not prevented the gradual disappearance of psychotherapy from the skill set of psychiatrists over the last decade.

In fact, the training of psychiatrists makes little sense. Why do we go to medical school? How do months of intensive training in surgery, internal medicine, radiology, etc., help psychiatrists treat mental illness? I've asked many of my colleagues if they thought medical school was useful for what they actually do as they sit in their offices talking to patients, and the common response is some version of "medical school is absolutely crucial, because I am constantly having to rule out medical conditions as I evaluate patients, I have to think about how the drugs I prescribe might interact with other drugs, and I have to monitor blood levels of drugs and possible side effects."

Being in the trenches myself, I agree that we do all these things and need to be trained to do them well. My argument is simply that we can learn all these things very well in a fraction of the time it takes to go through premed classes in college, four years of medical school, one year of medical internship, and three years of psychiatric residency. Why do I need to spend years perfecting the physical exam, learning surgery techniques, delivering babies, reading X-rays, and prescribing medications for nonpsychiatric illnesses, when in my professional life I will do none of these things? Do I really need medical school to recognize when to refer a patient to an internist or a neurologist? No, but I need to learn the skills of basic medical triage.

Do I need medical school to learn which labs to order when I prescribe certain drugs? No, but I need a good course in psychopharmacology and lab interpretation. Do I need medical school to learn the common side effects of drugs? No, but I need a course designed to teach me this knowledge.

Medical schools have changed over the years and now include courses on the importance of psychological factors in physical healing. But make no mistake—it is called "medical" school for a reason. Its purpose is to teach students how to combine patient interviews, physical exams, and laboratory tools to diagnose biomedical diseases, and then to combine advice, medications, and technical procedures to cure them. The basis for it all is an understanding of pathophysiology. But in psychiatry, we do not know the pathophysiology of mental illnesses, and therefore we do not use physical exams or laboratory data to diagnose.

Each year, the American Association of Medical Colleges summarizes and organizes the medical school performance of students by the specialty they end up choosing.[12] Future psychiatrists consistently rank at or near the bottom in all measures, including scores on both Part 1 and Part 2 of the medical board exams and the percentage of students qualifying for the medical student honor society, Alpha Omega Alpha. This is not because these students are dumb; rather, it reflects their accurate insight that most of the medical school curricula will be useless for their psychiatric careers. Therefore, they put less effort into mastering the material, and who can blame them?

In my opinion, medical school is the wrong place to train psychiatrists, for several reasons:

- It indoctrinates us into an excessively biomedical view of multidisciplinary problems.
- It gives us a feeling of inferiority among medical colleagues, because we are seen as being less medically competent.
- It simultaneously encourages in us a feeling of superiority among mental health professionals, as we wear our medi-

cal degrees as badges of honor to lord over those who are lower in the pecking order.

- It deprives us of precious time that we should use to learn skills and knowledge relevant to our work, such as different types of psychotherapies, family treatment, group treatment, neuropsychological assessment, and the use of community supports for chronic mental illness.

2. License all psychologists to become prescribers.

Licensing psychologists to become prescribers, unthinkable a decade ago, seems an increasingly realistic option. Prescribing psychologists are close to the ideal mental health professional, in that doctoral students specialize in understanding psychopathology, doing psychotherapy, and marshaling a range of psychosocial resources. On the other hand, simply tacking on a two-year intensive course in psychopharmacology at the end of such training is inefficient. It would be better to create programs that integrate psychopharmacology and psychological techniques from the very beginning of training.

3. Expand psychiatric nurse-practitioner training to enhance their competence.

As we've seen, NPs do a competent job treating psychiatric patients. The problem is that they have relatively little training in psychological approaches. During their basic nursing training, they rotate briefly through psychiatry inpatient units, and their two-year master's has to cram in training in both psychopharmacology *and* psychotherapy. That's a very tall order. Responding to this problem, the nursing associations are moving toward adding an additional year to NP training. But it seems highly doubtful that three years of postgraduate training will be enough to produce practitioners who can master all aspects of both medication and therapy treatment.

4. Build a new training program from the ground up.
For a span of fifteen years in the 1970s and 1980s, an intriguing training program flourished briefly in California, and here is the story of one of the trainees.

In 1973, Lawrence Gelb graduated from Harvard, and, like many newly minted college grads, was not certain what to do next. Gelb had majored in "social relations," an interdisciplinary department established by pioneering psychologist William James at Harvard at the turn of the century. "It was a combination of anthropology, psychology, and sociology," Gelb told me in an interview. He was interested in advanced psychology training of some sort, but he decided to test the waters first by taking a job at the Erich Lindemann Mental Health Center in Boston. There, his title was "therapeutic milieu leader." "Basically," he said, "I was a glorified mental health worker in the inpatient psychiatry unit. Most of the patients were schizophrenic and our main job was to get them stabilized on medication so they could go back into the community. The main drugs then were Haldol and Prolixin."

After two years, Gelb felt ready to move on. He considered a psychology PhD program, but he wasn't interested in the emphasis on research design and psychological testing. Psychiatry had appeal, but in order to get into medical school he would have had to go back to college to take the required premed courses, an unpleasant prospect.

Around then, he heard about a new training program that was just starting in the San Francisco Bay Area. Called the "Doctorate in Mental Health," it was a completely new five-year degree that was intended to be a hybrid of medical school and psychology graduate school. It was spearheaded by Dr. Robert Wallerstein, a famed psychoanalyst who would eventually become the chairman of the department of psychiatry at the University of California at San Francisco. Already, in the mid-seventies, Wallerstein sensed that psychiatry was abandoning psychotherapy, and the new degree was his effort to correct this.

The program consisted of two years of medical school classroom courses followed by three years of on-the-job training identical to a psychiatric residency. It was very similar to a regular program of medical school followed by residency, with the omission of two years of clinical rotations in nonpsychiatric medical specialties and the absence of the grueling one-year medical internship.

Gelb was admitted to the second class of the new program. During the classroom portion, which took place on the UC Berkeley campus, he took biochemistry, physiology, neuroanatomy, and other conventional medical school courses. But these were augmented by courses in psychoanalytic theory and social sciences. At UCSF, Gelb followed the same track as psychiatric residents. "We did all the same rotations in the inpatient units, the crisis unit, the adolescent unit, and we were on call in the ER."

In the end, Gelb felt that he had developed competence in prescribing psychiatric medications, but as it turned out, he and his classmates were never allowed to use these skills after graduation. Both the California Medical Society and the Northern California Psychiatric Society lobbied against a bill that would have licensed Gelb and his colleagues to prescribe psychotropic medicines in the state, and the bill was soundly defeated.

"The arguments against our program were couched in terms of safety, but they were not based on any empirical evidence that our training was not sound or that we made clinical mistakes—it was all about the underlying guild issues."

Ultimately, some of Gelb's classmates actually went to medical school and became psychiatrists. Gelb ended up getting a Harvard MBA and founded one of the nation's first health care advocacy companies, CareCounsel. Despite his substantial career successes, Gelb still looks back on his doctor of mental health degree with a sense of nostalgia and wistfulness. "All of us involved with the program felt it was the wave of the future—that this was the ideal way to train mental health professionals. It was a terrible thing, when the license was killed."

Does the doctor of mental health program offer a model for the psychiatrist of the future? Perhaps something like it should be resurrected. Two years of combined medical and psychological courses, followed by three years of psychiatric residency—it sounds sufficient, certainly more robust than a nurse practitioner's two or three years of training, and more efficient than adding two years on top of a PhD in psychology.

There's nothing quite like being a psychiatrist. Sometimes, as I sit talking to patients about what is most important to them, I have to pinch myself to realize that I am actually getting paid to do something that is so interesting and that is so helpful to people. But the question I have explored in this book is whether we are as helpful as we can be.

My job is to work with patients as they put together the pieces of their lives, whether through the biochemical salve of medication or the empathic give-and-take of psychotherapy. But sadly, psychiatry itself has become unhinged, fractured by scandals, by debates, and by the skepticism of an increasingly informed public. A recent Gallup poll found that only 38 percent of Americans believe that psychiatrists adhere to "high" or "very high" ethical standards. This puts psychiatrists on about the same level as bankers (37 percent) and chiropractors (36 percent). On the other hand, 69 percent rated physicians in general as trustworthy.[13]

As I write these words, the latest issue of *Psychiatric News*, the main periodical of the American Psychiatric Association, is lying on my desk. An article on the cover is headlined "Imaging, Genetics on Verge of Transforming Psychiatry." It waxes enthusiastic about genetic testing in psychiatry, vagus nerve stimulation, and similar topics.[14] Just below this article, also on the cover, appears the headline "Psychiatrist Helped Demonstrate Psychotherapy Is Cost-Effective," an item that profiles the work of Susan Lazar, a researcher who has devoted her life to studying the benefits of therapy.[15] These contrasting stories perfectly illustrate psychiatry's ongoing struggle to understand itself.

What kind of profession are we, and what should we become? Will we become psychoneurologists, forever chasing the latest "intriguing" brain findings in the hopes of interposing technology between us and our patients? Or will we become, as I advocate, psychological healers, returning to the basics of understanding our patients, and using machines, medications, and lab tests only when they clearly add something of value? Over the past two decades, psychiatry has gone astray. We have allowed our treatment decisions to be influenced by the promise of riches from drug companies, rather than by what our patients most need. We have fought pitched turf wars with our colleagues in related disciplines, instead of learning from them and incorporating their effective therapeutic tools into our own arsenals. Finally, we have unquestioningly sought to become just as "medical" as other doctors, when we should embrace the fact that psychiatry is remarkably different from the rest of medicine.

Recently, I started working with a new patient, Monica, who was abused by her father as a youngster. She is raising her own family now, and she came to me because she wants to avoid treating her children as she was treated. Unlike Carol, the woman whose story I told at the beginning of this book, I am doing both therapy and medication treatment for Monica. It isn't easy. I am spending extra time reading articles on state-of-the-art psychological treatments of PTSD. I am taking copious notes during our sessions in order to understand the links between the abuse she suffered and her current symptoms of insomnia, anxiety, and poor motivation. A few weeks ago, I asked her how her medication, Celexa, was working for her.

"It is definitely helping me function," she said. "But I still feel this tension anytime I need to tell my daughter to do something. I start to remember how scared I felt when my father raised his voice at me, and then I just stop talking. But I should be able to discipline my daughter appropriately. That's why I'm coming to therapy."

"Yes," I nodded, "this is definitely something we can work on. Tell me more about what you experience at those moments."

Monica talked, and I listened.

NOTES

Chapter 1: The Trouble with Psychiatry

1. Ramin Mojtabai and Mark Olfson, "National Trends in Psychotherapy by Office-Based Psychiatrists," *Archives of General Psychiatry* 65 (2008):962–970.

2. Alan F. Schatzberg and Charles B. Nemeroff, eds., *The American Psychiatric Publishing Textbook of Psychopharmacology* (Arlington, Va.: American Psychiatric Publishing, Inc., 2009).

3. Thomas R. Insel, "Translating Scientific Opportunity Into Public Health Impact: A Strategic Plan for Research on Mental Illness," *Archives of General Psychiatry* 66 (2) (2009):128–133.

4. David Foster Wallace, *Infinite Jest* (New York: Little, Brown, 1996).

5. D. T. Max, "The Unfinished," *The New Yorker*, March 9, 2009.

6. David Lipsky, "The Lost Years and Last Days of David Foster Wallace," *Rolling Stone*, posted October 30, 2008, http://www.rollingstone.com/news/story/23638511.

7. See Kitty Dukakis and Larry Tye, *Shock: The Healing Power of Electroconvulsive Therapy* (New York: Avery, 2006).

8. Each of these research projects focused on different psychiatric conditions. The CATIE trial (Clinical Antipsychotic Trials of Interventional Effectiveness) enrolled 1,600 patients with schizophrenia (http://www.catie.unc.edu/schizophrenia/synopsis.html); the STAR-D trial (Sequenced Treatment Alternatives to Relieve Depression) studied more than 4,000 patients with depression (see http://www.edc.pitt.edu/stard/); and the STEP-BD trial (Systematic Treatment Enhancement Program for Bipolar Disorder) enrolled more than 4,300 patients with bipolar disorder (see http://www.stepbd.org/).

9. Of the three antipsychotics listed, Zyprexa is the worst offender in terms of weight gain, causing as much as one pound of weight gain per week, while Seroquel and Risperdal are more moderate in their weight-gain liabilities. The FDA now requires that all makers of antipsychotics warn prescribers that their drugs may cause diabetes, although the data for this link is strongest for Zyprexa. Both obesity and diabetes are risk factors for heart disease. Thus far, it appears that the antipsychotics Geodon and Abilify are quite safe in terms of weight gain and diabetes, although they have other potential side effects, such as electrocardiogram abnormalities (Geodon) and agitation (Abilify). For a rank ordering of the diabetes

risks of the antipsychotics, see "Consensus Development Conference on Antipsychotic Drugs and Obesity and Diabetes," American Diabetes Association/American Psychiatric Association/American Association of Clinical Endocrinologists/North American Association for the Study of Obesity, *Diabetes Care*, (2004), 27(2):596–601.

10. Direct-to-consumer advertising figures (DTCA) are from the Sourcewatch website at http://www.sourcewatch.org/index.php?title=Direct-to-consumer_advertising_in_the_United_States and from Natasha Singer, "Lawmakers Seek to Curb Drug Commercials," *New York Times*, July 27, 2009, B1.

Chapter 2: On Becoming a Psychiatrist

1. New Mexico granted psychologists limited prescribing privileges in 2001, and Louisiana passed a similar law in 2004. Oregon is poised to adopt similar legislation.

2. The utility of ordering screening labs and brain imaging studies in psychiatry is debated to this day. Most studies have shown that the typical shotgun approach, in which psychiatrists order a standard list of tests for all new patients simply to "rule out" a hidden medical illness, leads to few clinically relevant results. For example, in one study 725 older depressed patients were given thyroid tests; only five patients (0.7% of the total) had abnormalities, and it was not clear that these abnormal values caused the depressive symptoms, or were simply accidental and unrelated findings. See Shelagh A. Fraser, Kurt Kroenke, et al., "Low Yield of Thyroid-Stimulating Hormone Testing in Elderly Patients with Depression," *General Hospital Psychiatry* 26 (2004):302–309.

3. Brief Psychotic Disorder is a diagnosis given to patients who present with at least one symptom of psychosis (such as delusions or hallucinations) but who have no past history of a significant psychiatric disorder. The psychosis is usually caused by severe stress, and the symptoms typically disappear within days or weeks. Schizophrenia, on the other hand, appears gradually over several years and develops into a chronic, long-term illness.

4. One of the classic books on narcissism is Heinz Kohut's *The Analysis of the Self: A Systematic Approach to the Psychoanalytic Treatment of Narcissistic Personality Disorders* (University of Chicago Press, 2009; original edition published by International Universities Press in 1971).

5. Ingeborg Van Pelt, "Where Is the Hurt? How Do We Help?" *Clinical Psychiatry News* 37 (6) (2009):10.

6. For an excellent technical survey of borderline personality disorder, see John Gunderson, *Borderline Personality Disorder: A Clinical Guide*, 2nd ed. (Arlington, Va.: American Psychiatric Publishing, Inc., 2008). For a layperson's guide, see Paul Mason, *Stop Walking on Eggshells: Taking Your Life Back When Someone You Care About Has Borderline Personality Disorder* (Oakland, Calif.: New Harbinger Publications, 1998).

7. For a description of dialectical behavioral therapy (a subtype of cognitive behavioral therapy), see Marsha Linehan, *Cognitive-Behavioral Treatment of Borderline Personality Disorder* (New York: Guilford Press, 1993).

8. The question of using medication or psychotherapy (or both) for treating borderline personality disorder continues to be debated in 2010. Most authorities, even those who acknowledge the value of medications, consider psychotherapy the first-line treatment for borderline personality disorder (see, for example, Joel Paris, *Treatment of Borderline Personality Disorder* [New York: Guilford Press, 2008]). The most effective therapies help patients to manage their chaotic emotions, decrease impulsivity, deal with imperfect relationships, and work on getting more structure into their lives. Medications work best when specifically targeted to psychiatric symptoms such as depression, impulsivity, or irrational thoughts (see Theo Ingenhoven, Patricia Lafay, et al., "Effectiveness of Pharmacotherapy for Severe Personality Disorders: Meta-Analyses of Randomized Controlled Trials," *Journal of Clinical Psychiatry* [pub. ahead of print]: (September 22, 2009); 71(1) (2010):14–25.

9. Temporal lobe epilepsy (TLE), also known as "complex partial seizures," is a legitimate neurological disorder, and several medications are FDA-approved for its treatment. The typical patients with TLE report a brief aura before the seizure, which may involve odd experiences such as déjà vu, hallucinated smells or tastes, or a sense that objects are much larger or much smaller than they are. After the aura, the actual seizure usually consists of a motionless stare in which patients either stop what they are doing or continue to perform simple actions mindlessly, as though they are robots. See the emedicine article "Temporal Lobe Epilepsy" for a good overview (http://emedicine.medscape.com/article/1184509-overview, accessed11/18/09). Dr. Murray and other faculty at MGH were proponents of the notion that TLE might underly the psychiatric symptoms of more patients than we realize; see, for example, Theodore Stern and George Murray, "Complex Partial Seizures Presenting as a Psychiatric Illness," *Journal of Nervous and Mental Disease* 172 (10) (1984):625–627.

Chapter 3: The Bible of Psychiatry

1. American Psychiatric Association, *Diagnostic and Statistical Manual of Mental Disorders, Fourth Ed., Text Revision* (Washington, D.C.: American Psychiatric Association, 2000). The current version of the DSM is called DSM-IV-TR, but for simplicity I have shortened it to DSM-IV, which was originally published in 1994. The diagnoses contained in the current "TR" version are identical to the 1994 version; the difference is that more explanatory text was added in 2000.

2. See chapter 9, "The Missing Skill," for a more extensive discussion of psychotherapy.

3. For historical facts on Emil Kraepelin, I relied largely on Edward Shorter, *A History of Psychiatry* (New York: John Wiley & Sons, Inc., 1997), 99–109.

4. I learned about Robert Spitzer from my interviews with him and from a fascinating published profile: Alix Spiegel, "The Dictionary of Disorder: How One Man Revolutionized Psychiatry," *The New Yorker*, January 3, 2005.

5. American Psychiatric Association, *Diagnostic and Statistical Manual of Mental Disorders, Second Ed.* (Washington, D.C.: American Psychiatric Association, 1968).

6. For a review of the poor diagnostic reliability of DSM-I and DSM-II, see Robert Spitzer, J.B. Forman, et al., "DSM-III Field Trials: I. Initial Interrater Diagnostic Reliability," *American Journal of Psychiatry* 136 (1979):815–817.

7. See John Feighner, Eli Robins, et al., "Diagnostic Criteria for Use in Psychiatric Research," *Archives of General Psychiatry* 26 (1972):57–63.

8. The two books referred to are: Herb Kutchins and Stuart Kirk, *The Selling of DSM: The Rhetoric of Science in Psychiatry* (Edison, N.J.: Aldine Transaction, 1992), and Herb Kutchins and Stuart Kirk, *Making Us Crazy* (New York: The Free Press, 1997). The quote is from *Making Us Crazy*, 28.

9. Ibid., 22.

10. Quoted in Benedict Carey, "Most Will Be Mentally Ill at Some Point, Study Says," *New York Times*, June 7, 2005.

11. This is a simplification of the full DSM-IV-TR criteria, which can be found in American Psychiatric Association, *Diagnostic and Statistical Manual of Mental Disorders, Fourth Ed., Text Revision, Desk Reference* (Washington, D.C.: American Psychiatric Association, 2000), 215. The full criteria include other specifications, the most crucial of which is that the distress interferes in some way with normal functioning.

12. Christopher Lane, *Shyness: How Normal Behavior Became a Sickness* (New Haven, Conn.: Yale University Press, 2007).

13. Ibid., 1

14. Premenstrual dysphoric disorder is classified as a subtype of "Depressive Disorder Not Otherwise Specified" in *DSM-IV-TR*, op. cit., 178.

15. Joan Chrisler and Paula Caplan, "The Strange Case of Dr. Jekyll and Ms. Hyde: How PMS Became a Cultural Phenomenon and Psychiatric Disorder," *Annual Review of Sex Research* 13 (2002):274–306.

16. Quoted in Jennifer Daw, "Is PMDD Real?" *APA Monitor on Psychology*, 33, no. 9, (2002), http://www.apa.org/monitor/oct02/pmdd.html.

17. David Kupfer, Michael First, and Darrel Regier, eds., *A Research Agenda for DSM-V* (Washington D.C.: American Psychiatric Association, 2002), xix.

18. Ibid.

19. Robert Spitzer, "DSM-V: Open and Transparent?" *Psychiatric News*, July 18, 2008, 43 (14):26.

20. Nada Stotland, James Scully, David Kupfer, and Darrel Regier, "DSM-V: Open and Transparent? Response," *Psychiatric News* 43 (14), July 18, 2008):26.

21. The DSM-V website, http://ww2.psych.org/MainMenu/Research/DSMIV/DSMV.aspx, is open to the public.

22. Allen Frances, "A Warning Sign on the Road to *DSM-V*: Beware of Its Unintended Consequences," *Psychiatric Times*, June 26, 2009.

23. For a copy of Dr. Costello's resignation letter, see the July 7, 2009, posting on The Carlat Psychiatry Blog, http://carlatpsychiatry.blogspot.com/2009/07/dsm-v-armageddon-part-2.html.

24. Alan Schatzberg, James Scully, David Kupfer, and Darrel Regier, "Setting the Record Straight: A Response to Frances Commentary on DSM-V," *Psychiatric Times*, July 1, 2009.

25. Alex Beam, "Who's Crazy Now?" *Boston Globe*, July 17, 2009.

26. Darrel Regier, interview by author, December 19, 2008.

27. For a review of mild cognitive impairment, see Paul Rosenberg, Deirdre Johnston, et al., "A Clinical Approach to Mild Cognitive Impairment," *American Journal of Psychiatry* 163 (11) (2006):1884–1890.

28. Howard Feldman and Claudia Jacova, "Mild Cognitive Impairment," *American Journal of Geriatric Psychiatry* 13 (2005):645–655.

29. Rachelle Doody, Steven Ferris, et al., "Donepezil Treatment of Patients with MCI: A 48-Week Randomized, Placebo-Controlled Trial," *Neurology* 72 (2009), 1555–61.

30. See http://www.rxlist.com/paxil-drug.htm for a list of FDA-approved indications for Paxil.

Chapter 4: How Medications Became the New Therapy

1. David Healy, *The Anti-Depressant Era* (Cambridge, Mass.: Harvard University Press, 1997), 13.

2. Mark Olfson and Steven Marcus, "National Patterns in Antidepressant Medication Treatment," *Archives of General Psychiatry* 66(8) (2009):848–856.

3. Ben Harder, "Sleep Treatments Rise to the Occasion," *USA Today*, posted 2/26/06, http://www.usatoday.com/news/health/2006-02-26-sleep-treatments_x.htm.

4. University of Florida, "UF study examines heart risks of stimulants in children with ADHD," posted December 3, 2007, http://news.ufl.edu/2007/12/03/uf-study-examines-heart-risks-of-stimulants-in-children-with-adhd/.

5. U.S. Food and Drug Administration, "FDA Requests Label Change for All Sleep Disorder Drug Products," news release, March 14, 2007, http://www.fda.gov/NewsEvents/Newsroom/PressAnnouncements/2007/ucm108868.htm.

6. For a popular textbook of neuroscience used by psychiatrists, see Stephen Stahl, *Stahl's Essential Psychopharmacology* (New York: Cambridge University Press, 2008).

7. For a critical review of the monoamine hypothesis, see Eero Castrén, "Is Mood Chemistry?" *Nature Reviews Neuroscience* 6 (2005):241–246.

8. R. H. Belmaker and Galila Agam, "Major Depressive Disorder," *New England Journal of Medicine* 358 (2008):55–68.

9. Linda Booij, Willem Van der Does, et al., "Monoamine Depletion in Psychiatric and Healthy Populations: Review," *Molecular Psychiatry* 8 (2003):951–973.

10. J. Moncrieff, "A Critique of the Dopamine Hypothesis of Schizophrenia and Psychosis," *Harvard Review of Psychiatry* 17 (2009):214–225.

11. James Maas, Charles Bowden, et al., "Schizophrenia, Psychosis, and Cerebral Spinal Fluid Homovanillic Acid Concentrations," *Schizophrenia Bulletin* 23 (1997):147–154.

12. Dost Ongur, "Topics in the Treatment of Schizophrenia," *The Carlat Psychiatry Report* 7 (12) (2009):4.

13. Matcheri Keshavan, Rajiv Tandon, et al., "Schizophrenia, 'Just the Facts': What We Know in 2008: Part 3: Neurobiology," *Schizophrenia Research* 106 (2008):89–107.

14. One of the most prominent such companies is 23 and Me. On their Web site, they list 47 conditions and traits covered by their $429 health information genetic kit: https://www.23andme.com/health/all/.

15. Avshalom Caspi, Karen Sugden, et al., "Influence of Life Stress on Depression: Moderation by a Polymorphism in the 5-HTT Gene," *Science* 301 (2003):386–389.

16. Neil Risch, Richard Herrell, et al., "Interaction Between the Serotonin Transporter Gene (5-HTTLPR), Stressful Life Events, and Risk of Depression: A Meta-analysis," *Journal of the American Medical Association* 301 (2009):2462–2471.

17. Quoted in Robert Langreth, "Hunt for Depression Genes Goes into Reverse," *Forbes*, posted June 16, 2009, http://www.forbes.com/2009/06/16/depression-genetics-jama-business-healthcare-genes_print.html.

18. Nancy Andreasen, *Brave New Brain: Conquering Mental Illness in the Era of the Genome* (Oxford, U.K.: Oxford University Press, 2001).

19. The main results: Hreinn Stefansson, Roel A. Ophoff, et al., "Common Variants Conferring Risk of Schizophrenia," *Nature* 460 (2009):744–747.

20. Nicholas Wade, "Hoopla, and Disappointment in Schizophrenia Research," TierneyLab Blog, *New York Times*, posted July 1, 2009, http://tierneylab.blogs.nytimes.com/2009/07/01/hoopla-and-disappointment-in-schizophrenia-research/?hpw.

21. Jeffrey Lacasse and Jonathan Leo, "Serotonin and Depression: A Disconnect Between the Advertisements and the Scientific Literature," *PLoS Medicine*, (12) (2005):e392.

22. American Psychiatric Association, *Practice Guideline for the Treatment of Patients with Major Depressive Disorder, 2nd ed.* (2000), 21, available online at http://www.psychiatryonline.com/pracGuide/pracGuideChapToc_7.aspx.

23. A. John Rush, Madhukar Trivedi, et al., "Bupropion-SR, Sertraline, or Venlafaxine-XR After Failure of SSRIs for Depression," *New England Journal of Medicine* 354 (2006):1231–1242.

24. Edward Shorter, *A History of Psychiatry* (New York: John Wiley & Sons, Inc., 1997), 99–109.

25. Kay Redfield Jamison, *An Unquiet Mind* (New York: Knopf, 1996), 67.

26. John Cade, "Lithim Salts in the Treatment of Psychotic Excitement," *Medical Journal of Australia* 2 (September 3, 1949):349–352.

27. See both David Healy, *Let Them Eat Prozac* (New York: New York University Press, 2004), and Joseph Glenmullen, *Prozac Backlash* (New York: Simon & Schuster, 2001).

28. For a thorough review of the data on antidepressants and sexuality, see Richard Balon, "Depression, Antidepressants, and Human Sexuality," *Primary Psychiatry* 14 (2) (2007):42–50.

29. Antonei Csoka, Audrey Bahrick, et al., "Persistent Sexual Dysfunction After Discontinuation of Selective Serotonin Reuptake Inhibitors," *Journal of Sexual Medicine* 5 (2008):227–233.

30. Martin Teicher, Carol Glod, et al., "Emergence of intense suicidal preoccupation during fluoxetine treatment," *American Journal of Psychiatry* 147 (1990):207–210.

31. Gardiner Harris, "F.D.A. Panel Urges Stronger Warning on Antidepressants," *New York Times*, posted September 15, 2004, http://www.nytimes.com/2004/09/15/health/15depress.html.

32. David Fassler, "Antidepressants and Suicidal Ideation," *The Carlat Psychiatry Report* 6(11) (2008):4.

33. Andrew Leon, "The Revised Warning for Antidepressants and Suicidality: Unveiling the Black Box of Statistical Analyses," *American Journal of Psychiatry* 164 (December 2007): 1786–1789.

34. Thomas Laughren, "Overview for December 13 Meeting of Psychopharmacology Drugs Advisory Committee," available online at http://www.fda.gov.ezproxy.library.tufts.edu/OHRMS/DOCKETS/AC/06/briefing/2006-4272b1-01-FDA.pdf, accessed November 25, 2009.

35. Mark Olfson, Steven Marcus, et al., "Effects of Food and Drug Administration Warnings on Antidepressant Use in a National Sample," *Archives of General Psychiatry* 65(1) (2008):94–101.

36. Robert Gibbons, Kwan Hur, et al., "The Relationship Between Antidepressant Prescription Rates and Rate of Early Adolescent Suicide; *American Journal of Psychiatry* 163(11) (2006):1898–1904.

Chapter 5: How Companies Sell Psychiatrists on Their Drugs

1. Most of the material on the marketing tactics used for promoting Neurontin are documented in Melody Peterson, *Our Daily Meds* (New York: Farrar, Straus, and Giroux/Sarah Crichton Books, 2008), 212–252.

2. United States Government Accountability Office, New Drug Development, November 2006. Available online at http://www.gao.gov/new.items/d0749.pdf.

3. Quoted in American Society of Health-Systems Pharmacists, "Drug Innovation on the Decline," *AJHP News*, February 1, 2007.

4. Several excellent books have profiled the increasingly deceptive marketing tactics of the pharmaceutical industry and have been invaluable sources for me in researching this book. These include Marcia Angell, *The Truth About the Drug Companies* (New York: Random House, 2004); John Abramson, *Overdosed America* (New York: HarperCollins, 2004); Jerome Kassirer, *On the Take* (Oxford, U.K., Oxford University Press, 2005); and Alison Bass, *Side Effects* (Chapel Hill, N.C.: Algonquin Books, 2008).

5. Erick Turner, Annette M. Matthews, et. al., "Selective Publication of Antidepressant Trials and Its Influence on Apparent Efficacy," *New England Journal of Medicine* 358 (2008):252–60 (see chart on p. 257 for data I cited on Celexa).

6. Andrea Cipriani, Toshiaki Furukawa, et al., "Comparative Efficacy and Acceptability of 12 New-Generation Antidepressants: A Multiple-Treatments Meta-Analysis," *Lancet* 373 (2009):746–758.

7. Gardiner Harris, "Research Center Tied to Drug Company" *New York Times*, November 25, 2008, A22.

8. Quoted in Merrill Goozner, *The $800 Million Pill* (University of California Press, 2005).

9. Marc-Andre Gagnon and Joel Lexchin, "The Cost of Pushing Pills: A New Estimate of Pharmaceutical Promotion Expenditures in the United States," *PLoS Medicine* 5 (1) (2008):e1 doi:10.1371/journal.pmed.0050001.

10. Public Citizen, "2002 Drug Industry Profits: Hefty Pharmaceutical Company Margins Dwarf Other Industries," *Congress Watch Report*, June 2003, online at http://www.citizen.org/documents/Pharma_Report.pdf.

11. Eli Lilly news release, "Lilly Reports Fourth-Quarter and Full-Year 2008 Results," posted January 29, 2009, http://newsroom.lilly.com/ReleaseDetail.cfm?releaseid=362195.

12. See Wikinvest/Wyeth webpage, http://www.wikinvest.com/stock/Wyeth_%28WYE%29.

13. Catherine Larkin, "Forest's Third-Quarter Profit Increases on Drug Sales (Update 6)" Bloomberg.com, posted January 15, 2008, http://www.bloomberg.com/apps/news?pid=20601103&sid=aH_tYyGgTofM&refer=us.

14. Adriane Fugh-Berman and Shahram Ahari, "Following the Script: How Drug Reps Make Friends and Influence Doctors," *PLoS Medicine* 4 (4) (2007):e150 . doi:10.1371/journal.pmed.0040150.

15. Jeanne Lenzer, "Confessions of a Drug Rep" (movie review), *British Medical Journal* 330 (April 16, 2005):911: doi:10.1136/bmj.330.7496.911.

16. For a full account of my year as a speaker for Wyeth, see Daniel Carlat, "Dr. Drug Rep," *New York Times Magazine*, November 25, 2007, http://www.nytimes.com/2007/11/25/magazine/25memoir-t.html.

17. Ashley Wazana, "Physicians and the Pharmaceutical Industry: Is a Gift Ever Just a Gift?" *Journal of the American Medical Association* 283 (2000):373–380.

18. Jason Dana and George Loewenstein, "A Social Science Perspective on Gifts to Physicians," *Journal of the American Medical Association* 290 (2) (2003).

19. Wallace Mendelson, "A Review of the Evidence for the Efficacy and Safety of Trazodone in Insomnia," *Journal of Clinical Psychiatry* 66 (4) (April 2005):469–76.

20. Daniel Carlat, "Generic Smear Campaign," *New York Times*, May 9, 2006, op-ed page.

21. David Healy and Dinah Cattell, "Interface Between Authorship, Industry, and Science in the Domain of Therapeutics," *The British Journal of Psychiatry* 183 (2003):22–27.

22. Joel Lexchin and Lisa Bero, "Pharmaceutical Industry Sponsorship and Research Outcome and Quality: Systematic Review," *British Medical Journal* 326 (7400) (May 31, 2003):1167.

23. Erick Turner, Annette M. Matthews, et. al., "Selective Publication of Antidepressant Trials and Its Influence on Apparent Efficacy," *New England Journal of Medicine* 358 (2008):252–60.

24. Erick Turner, interview with author.

25. Mark Zimmerman, J. Mattia, and Michael Posternak, "Are Subjects in Pharmacological Treatment Trials of Depression Representative of Patients in Routine Clinical Practice?" *American Journal of Psychiatry* 159(3) (March 1, 2002):469–73.

26. Alan Finder, "Elite Colleges Reporting Record Lows in Admission," *New York Times*, April 1, 2008.

27. C. D. DeAngelis, J. M. Drazen, F. A. Frizelle, et al., "Clinical Trial Registration: A Statement from the International Committee of Medical Journal Editors," *Journal of the American Medical Association* 292 (2004):1363–1364.

28. Matthew Perrone, "States Fight to Shield Docs from Drug Data Mining," *Boston Globe*, August 19, 2008.

29. Louis Porter, "Data Mining Hearing Refused," *Rutland Herald*, June 30, 2009.

30. Pharmaceutical Research and Manufacturers of America, *Code on Interactions with Healthcare Professionals*, January 2009, online at http://www.phrma.org/files/PhRMA%20Marketing%20Code%202008.pdf.

Chapter 6: The Hired Guns

1. Two states, Vermont and Minnesota, have publicly disclosed drug company payments to physicians, and in both states psychiatrists received the most money. In addition, in Eli Lilly's recently disclosed list of physician payments, of twenty-two doctors receiving $50,000 to $70,000 during the first quarter of 2009, fifteen were psychiatrists (see "Lilly Outside 'Faculty' Is Headed by 22 Physicians Receiving $50,000 or More," *The Pink Sheet*, October 28, 2009).

2. For the full account, see Daniel Carlat, "Dr. Drug Rep," *New York Times Magazine*, November 25, 2007, online at http://www.nytimes.com/2007/11/25/magazine/25memoir-t.html.

3. Michael Thase and Richard Entsuah, "Remission rates during treatment with venlafaxine or selective serotonin reuptake inhibitors," *The British Journal of Psychiatry* 178 (March 2001):234–241.

4. Jeremy Kassirer, interview with the author. Dr. Kassirer has expanded on these ideas in his book *On the Take* (Oxford, U.K.: Oxford University Press, 2005), which is the definitive indictment of hired-gun physicians.

5. Eric Campbell and Russell L. Gruen, "A National Survey of Physician-Industry Relationships," *New England Journal of Medicine* 356 (2007):1742–1750.

6. Kevin O'Reilly, "Doctors Increasingly Close Doors to Drug Reps, While Pharma Cuts Ranks," *American Medical News*, March 23, 2009.

7. As interviewed in Ray Moynihan, "Key Opinion Leaders: Independent Experts or Drug Representatives in Disguise?" *British Medical Journal* 336 (2008):1402–1403.

8. Scott Hensley and Barbara Martinez, "To Sell Their Drugs, Companies Increasingly Rely on Doctors," *Wall Street Journal*, July 15, 2005.

9. Giovanni Fava, "Should the Drug Industry Work with Key Opinion Leaders? No," *British Medical Journal* 336 (June 21, 2008):1405.

10. Michael Thase, "Effects of Venlafaxine on Blood Pressure: A Meta-Analysis of Original Data from 3,744 Depressed Patients," *Journal of Clinical Psychiatry* 59 (10) (October 2008):502–508.

11. Gardiner Harris, Benedict Carey, and Janet Roberts, "Psychiatrists, Children, and Drug Industry's Role," *New York Times*, May 10, 2007.

12. Gardiner Harris, "Lawmaker Calls for Registry of Drug Firms Paying Doctors," *New York Times*, August 4, 2007.

13. One of the fascinating back stories of Grassley's investigations is the role played by Paul Thacker, a former investigative reporter who joined the senator's staff. See the thoughtful article in *Nature* for a profile of Thacker: Meredith Wadman, "The Senator's Sleuth," *Nature* 461 (September 17, 2009):330–334.

14. Floor Statement of U.S. Senator Chuck Grassley of Iowa, "Pharma Payments to Doctors," Wednesday, April 2, 2008, online at http://finance.senate.gov/press/Gpress/2008/prg040208b.pdf.

15. Gardiner Harris and Benedict Carey, "Researchers Fail to Reveal Full Drug Pay," *New York Times*, June 8, 2008.

16. James Vaznis, "3 Psychiatrists Accused of Missteps Face Inquiry," *Boston Globe*, June 10, 2008.

17. Benedict Carey and Gardiner Harris, "Psychiatric Group Faces Scrutiny over Drug Industry Ties," *New York Times*, July 12, 2008.

18. Stanford University, Office of University Communications, "University Statement on Senator Grassley's June 23 Letter on Conflicts of Interest in Medical Research," posted June 25, 2008, http://ucomm.stanford.edu/news/062508conflict_of_interest.html.

19. Ed Silverman, "Who's In Charge? A Stanford Prof and an NIH Grant," Pharmalot blog, July 30, 2008, http://www.pharmalot.com/2008/07/whos-in-charge-a-stanford-prof-an-nih-grant/.

20. Grassley is quoted in Devin Banerjee, "Stanford Prof. Leaves Post Amid Senate Investigation into Ties to the Drug Industry" *Stanford Daily*, August 14, 2008.

21. Dr. Schatzberg's resignation as head of the NIMH grant was made public via a July 31, 2008, letter from Stanford University to Senator Grassley, which can be accessed online at http://ucomm.stanford.edu/news/073108_grassley.pdf.

22. James LaRossa and Genevieve Romano, "Boss of Bosses," *TEN: Trends in Evidence-Based Neuropsychiatry* 2(9) (September 2000).

23. Material in this section on Dr. Nemeroff is from various sources, particularly Gardiner Harris, "Top Psychiatrist Didn't Report Drug Makers' Pay," *New York Times*, October 3, 2008; the blog Health Care Renewal, especially a series of articles by Bernard Carroll focusing on Dr. Nemeroff; and sources as referenced below.

24. Charles Nemeroff, Helen S. Mayberg, et al., "VNS Therapy in Treatment-Resistant Depression: Clinical Evidence and Putative Neurobiological Mechanisms," *Neuropsychopharmacology* 31 (July 2006):1345–1355. Published online April 19, 2006, doi:10.1038/sj.npp.1301082.

25. David Armstrong, "Charles Nemeroff Steps Down Over Undisclosed Ties," *Wall Street Journal*, August 28, 2006.

26. Quoted in Craig Schneider, "Controversial Emory Researcher Leaving," *Atlanta Journal-Constitution*, October 30, 2009.

27. Kate Borger, "Nemeroff Accepts Offer at U. Miami," *Emory Wheel*, November 20, 2009.

28. Quoted in Valerie Bauman, "Ethics Questions Arise as Doctors Pitch to Colleagues," *USA Today*, March 8, 2008.

29. Howard Brody, *Hooked: Ethics, the Medical Profession, and the Pharmaceutical Industry* (Lanham, Md.: Rowman and Littlefield, 2007), 32.

30. Quoted in Gardiner Harris and Benedict Carey, "Researchers Fail to Reveal Full Drug Pay," *New York Times*, June 8, 2008.

Chapter 7: A Frenzy of Diagnosis

1. Maria Cramer and Raja Mishra, "Girl Fed Fatal Overdoses, Court Told," *Boston Globe*, February 7, 2007.

2. "DSS Timeline on Rebecca Riley," *Boston Globe*, February 8, 2007.

3. John Kelly, "Medical Board Lifts Sanction Against Doctor in Rebecca Riley Case," *Patriot Ledger*, September 12, 2009.

4. Scott Allen, "Backlash on Bipolar Diagnoses in Children," *Boston Globe*, June 17, 2007.

5. From Massachusetts General Hospital, Pediatric Psychopharmacology Department Web page, http://www2.massgeneral.org/allpsych/pedipsych/staff/biederman.html, accessed November 27, 2009.

6. See Source Watch article on Joseph Biederman, at http://www.sourcewatch.org/index.php?title=Joseph_Biederman.

7. Carey Goldberg, "Doctor Scrutinized for Drug-firm Ties Gets Kudos from Bipolar Patients, Kin," *Boston Globe*, January 30, 2009.

8. Allen, "Backlash on Bipolar Diagnoses in Children."

9. Gardiner Harris, "Drug Maker Told Studies Would Aid It, Papers Say," *New York Times*, March 19, 2009.

10. Lawrence Diller, "Misguided Standards of Care," *Boston Globe*, June 19, 2007, op-ed piece.

11. Joseph Biederman, Stephen Faraone, et al., "Attention-Deficit Hyperactivity Disorder and Juvenile Mania: An Overlooked Comorbidity?" *Journal of the American Academy of Child and Adolescent Psychiatry* 35(8) (August 1996):997–1008.

12. Henry Nasrallah, Donald Black, et al. "Diagnosing and Managing Psychotic and Mood Disorders," *Current Psychiatry* 7 (12S) (December 2008):S1–S31.

13. For a thorough and balanced review of the controversies regarding bipolar disorder in children, see Mani Pavuluri, Boris Birmaher, et al., "Pediatric Bipolar Disorder: A Review of the Past 10 Years," *Journal of the American Academy of Child and Adolescent Psychiatry* 44(9) (2005):846–871. For a less technical article, see Daniel Carlat, "Bipolar Disorder in Children: Is the Diagnosis Valid?" *The Carlat Psychiatry Report* 4 (8), (August 2006):1–2.

14. C. Moreno, G. Laje, et al, "National Trends in the Outpatient Diagnosis and Treatment of Bipolar Disorder in Youth," *Archives of General Psychiatry* 64 (2009):1032–1039.

15. Jennifer Harris, "The Increased Diagnosis of 'Juvenile Bipolar Disorder': What Are We Treating?" *Psychiatric Services* 56 (May 2005):529–531.

16. Massachusetts General Hospital Web site, "MGH Department of Psychiatry, Department Facts," accessed November 26, 2009, from http://www2.massgeneral.org/allpsych/facts1.asp.

17. Risperdal is now FDA-approved for the treatment of bipolar disorder in children and adolescents; Zyprexa is not yet approved, but it is expected to win approval.

18. Mauricio Tohen, Ludmila Kryzhanovskaya, et al., "Olanzapine versus Placebo in the Treatment of Adolescents with Bipolar Mania," *American Journal of Psychiatry* 164(10) (October 2007):1547–1556.

19. Gardiner Harris, "Research Center Tied to Drug Company," *New York Times*, November 25, 2008, A22.

20. "Credibility Crisis in Pediatric Psychiatry," *Nature Neuroscience* 11 (9) (September 11, 2008):983.

21. Charles Bradley, "The Behavior of Children Receiving Benzedrine," *American Journal of Psychiatry* 94 (November 1937):577–585.

22. Michael Smith, "Cardiovascular Safety Warning Added for Stimulants for ADHD," *MedPage Today*, August 23, 2006, http://www.medpagetoday.com/Psychiatry/ADHD-ADD/3987.

23. Stephen Faraone, Joseph Biederman, et al., "Effect of Stimulants on Height and Weight: A Review of the Literature," *Journal of the American Academy of Child and Adolescent Psychiatry* 47(9) (September 2008):994–1009.

24. Figures from Steven Nissen, "ADHD Drugs and Cardiovascular Risk," *New England Journal of Medicine* 354 (14) (2006):1445–1448.

25. Daniel Carlat, "Computerized Testing for ADHD: Is it Useful?" *The Carlat Psychiatry Report* 6(5) (2008):1–6.

26. Jennifer Setlik, G. Randall Bond, et al., "Adolescent Prescription ADHD Medication Abuse Is Rising Along With Prescriptions for These Medications," *Pediatrics* (August 24, 2004) [Epub ahead of print]; 124 (3)(September 2009):875–880.

27. For a detailed description of these Shire-funded newsletters, along with images, see "Announcing the 'Doctors for Dollars' Award," The Carlat Psychiatry Blog, June 25, 2007, at http://carlatpsychiatry.blogspot.com/2007/06/announcing-doctors-for-dollars-award.html.

28. Bill Alpert, "The Squeeze on Drug-Maker Shire," *Barron's Online*, June 20, 2008.

29. Lawrence Diller, *Running on Ritalin* (New York: Bantam Books, 1998), and *The Last Normal Child* (Westport, Conn.: Praeger, 2006).

30. Thomas Phelan, *1-2-3 Magic: Effective Discipline for Children 2-12*, 2nd ed. (Child Management, 1996).

31. Christian Teter, Sean Esteban McCabe, et al., "Illicit Use of Specific Prescription Stimulants Among College Students: Prevalence, Motives, and Routes of Administration," *Pharmacotherapy* 26(10) (2006):1501–1510.

32. Henry Greely, Barbara Sahakian, et al., "Towards Responsible Use of Cognitive-Enhancing Drugs by the Healthy," *Nature* 456 (December 10, 2008):702–705.

33. Brendan Maher, "Poll Results: Look Who's Doping," *Nature* 452 (2008): 674–675.

Chapter 8: The Seductions of Technology

1. For the history of electroconvulsive therapy, see both Edward Shorter and David Healy, *Shock Therapy* (New Brunswick, N.J.: Rutgers University Press, 2007),

and Edward Shorter, *A History of Psychiatry* (New York: John Wiley & Sons, Inc., 1997).

2. Ken Kesey, *One Flew over the Cuckoo's Nest* (New York: Signet, 1962).

3. U.S. Department of Health and Human Services. *Mental Health: A Report of the Surgeon General* (Rockville, Md.: U.S. Department of Health and Human Services, National Institute of Mental Health, 1999).

4. Figures on rates of ECT are from Massachusetts General Hospital Hotline Online, "Electroconvulsive Therapy Discussion Hosted at the MGH," October 13, 2006, http://www2.massgeneral.org/pubaffairs/issues2006/101306ect.htm.

5. Julie Lawrence, Position Statement, www.ect.org.

6. For a recent review of all ECT research, see Sarah H. Lisanby, "Electroconvulsive Therapy for Depression," *New England Journal of Medicine* 357 (2007):1939–1945.

7. James Potash, "A Shockingly Effective Treatment for Depression," ABC News Essay, January 29, 2008, http://abcnews.go.com/Health/Depression/story?id=4199997&page=1.

8. Charles Kellner, Rebecca Knapp, et al., "Continuation Electroconvulsive Therapy vs. Pharmacotherapy for Relapse Prevention in Major Depression," *Archives of General Psychiatry* 63 (2006):1337–1344.

9. For information and photos from the manufacturer of the vagus nerve stimulator, see their Web site at http://www.vnstherapy.com/depression/main.asp. VNS has been approved by the FDA for adjunctive treatment of epilepsy since 1997, and its effectiveness for this indication is widely accepted.

10. Gardiner Harris, "Device Won Approval Though F.D.A. Staff Objected," *New York Times*, February 17, 2006.

11. John Rush, Laura Marangell, et al. "Vagus Nerve Stimulation for Treatment-Resistant Depression: A Randomized, Controlled Acute Phase Trial." *Biological Psychiatry* 58 (2005):347–354.

12. Mark George, John Rush, et al., "A One-Year Comparison of Vagus Nerve Stimulation with Treatment as Usual for Treatment-Resistant Depression," *Biological Psychiatry* 58 (2005):364–373.

13. For the most thorough account of the sequence of events leading to the approval of VNS, see the Senate Finance Committee's report: Committee on Finance, *United States Senate: Review of the FDA's Approval Process for the Vagus Nerve Stimulation Therapy System for Treatment-Resistant Depression*, U.S. Government Printing Office, Washington, D.C., 2006. The full senate report is available online at http://finance.senate.gov/press/Gpress/02_2006%20report.pdf.

14. The testimony of Charles Donovan can be found in the transcript of the advisory meeting: Neurological Devices Panel of the Medical Devices Advisory Committee, Tuesday, June 15, 2004, online at http://www.fda.gov/ohrms/DOCKETS/ac/04/transcripts/Pages%20from%202004-4047t1-01.pdf.

15. Charles E. Donovan III, *Out of the Black Hole: The Patient's Guide to Vagus Nerve Stimulation and Depression* (St. Louis, Mo.: Wellness Publishers, LLC, 2005).

16. Robert Steyer, "Cyberonics CEO Seeing Red," The Street.com, posted 5/19/05,athttp://www.thestreet.com/story/10224416/1/cyberonics-ceo-seeing-red.html.

17. Public Citizen, "Approval of Device to Treat Depression Is One of Most Questionable FDA Decisions in Recent Memory," statement of Peter Lurie, M.D., M.P.H., deputy director, Public Citizen's Health Research Group, July 18, 2005, http://www.commondreams.org/news2005/0718-11.htm.

18. PRNewswire-FirstCall, press release, "Cyberonics Provides Update on Annual American Psychiatric Association Meeting Activities and Recent VNS Therapy Publications," posted Friday, May 19, 2006, http://www.redorbit.com/news/health/510939/cyberonics_provides_update_on_annual_american_psychiatric_association_meeting_activities/index.html.

19. A. John Rush, "Interpreting the Star-D Trial," *The Carlat Psychiatry Report* 4 (5) (2006):4–5.

20. Arif Khan, Nick Redding, et al., "The Persistence of the Placebo Response in Antidepressant Clinical Trials," *Journal of Psychiatric Research* 42 (10) (August 2004):791–796.

21. Miriam Shuchman, "Approving the Vagus-Nerve Stimulator for Depression," *New England Journal of Medicine* 356 (2007):1604–1607.

22. Centers for Medicare and Medicaid Services (CMS), Pub 100-03 Medicare National Coverage Determinations, Vagus Nerve Stimulation (VNS) for Resistant Depression, June 22, 2007, at http://www.cms.hhs.gov/Transmittals/Downloads/R70NCD.pdf.

23. Insulin coma therapy, also known as insulin shock therapy, was for years a standard treatment for schizophrenia and was practiced through the 1960s in more than 100 psychiatric hospitals in the United States. It was likely ineffective, and carried a mortality rate of at least 1 percent. Ironically, Manfred Sakel, who discovered the treatment, received the Nobel Prize for Medicine in 1957, shortly before insulin therapy was discredited (see Edward Shorter, *A History of Psychiatry* [New York: John Wiley and Sons, Inc., 1997], 207–215).

24. The transorbital prefrontal lobotomy was pioneered by Walter Freeman, primarily for the treatment of schizophrenia. The procedure took as little as five minutes, and involved hammering a pick through the bones above the eyeball and sweeping brain tissue away. Over 20,000 of the procedures were done in the United States through the 1950s. Eventually, a controlled study found that it was no more effective than no treatment (for the definitive history, see Jack El-Hai, *The Lobotomist* [Hoboken, N.J.: John Wiley and Sons, 2005]).

25. The bizarre surgical technique was practiced by Henry Cotton, a psychiatrist and medical director of the New Jersey State Hospital at Trenton from 1907 to 1930. Cotton believed that psychosis was caused by infections, and experimented with removing teeth from schizophrenic patients. In cases where this was not effective, he moved on to removing other organs, including tonsils, gall bladders, testicles, and ovaries. Mortality rates were up to 45 percent, and there is no evidence the technique was effective. See Andrew Scull, *Madhouse: A Tragic Tale of Megalomania and Modern Medicine* (New Haven, Conn.: Yale University Press, 2007).

26. For background on Mesmer, see "Franz Mesmer," Wikipedia: The Free Encyclopedia, http://en.wikipedia.org/wiki/Franz_Mesmer.

27. See the Mary Baker Eddy Library, "Timeline," http://www.marybakereddylibrary.org/mary-baker-eddy/timeline.

28. For official information from Neuronetics, the manufacturer of the only FDA-approved TMS device, see http://www.neuronetics.com/Home.aspx.

29. John O'Reardon, H. Brent Solvason, et al., "Efficacy and Safety of Transcranial Magnetic Stimulation in the Acute Treatment of Major Depression: A Multisite Randomized Controlled Trial," *Biological Psychiatry* 62 (11) (2007):1208–1216.

30. Sarah Lisanby, Mustafa Husain, et al., "Daily Left Prefrontal Repetitive Transcranial Magnetic Stimulation in the Acute Treatment of Major Depression: Clinical Predictors of Outcome in a Multisite, Randomized Controlled Clinical Trial," *Neuropsychopharmacology* 34 (2004):522–534.

31. See Lindner Center of Hope Web site: http://www.lindnercenterofhope.org/PatientCare/TMSTherapy/tabid/561/Default.aspx.

32. Neuronetics Press Release, "NeuroStar® TMS Therapy Improved Quality of Life in Patients with Major Depression in Clinical Trials," May 21, 2007, http://www.prnewswire.com/news-releases/neurostarr-tms-therapy-improved-quality-of-life-in-patients-with-major-depression-in-clinical-trials-58385412.html.

33. *Brain SPECT: Participate in the Imaging Revolution in Psychiatry*, brochure sent to author's office, October 2007.

34. For information on the Amen clinics, including locations, services offered, and books and other products sold by Dr. Amen, see his Web site: http://www.amenclinics.com/. The price of $3,300 for an evaluation was accurate as of December 2007, which is when I visited his clinic.

35. Daniel Amen, *Change Your Brain, Change Your Life* (New York: Three Rivers Press, 1999), and *Making a Good Brain Great* (New York: Three Rivers Press, 2006).

36. Harriet Hall, "A Skeptical View of SPECT Scans and Dr. Daniel Amen," Quackwatch, November 15, 2007, http://www.quackwatch.org/06ResearchProjects/amen.html.

37. As quoted in Paul Raeburn, "The Therapeutic Mind Scan," *New York Times*, February 20, 2005.

38. Daniel Carlat, "Brain Scans as Mind Readers? Don't Believe the Hype," *Wired*, June 2008.

39. American Psychiatric Association, Psychiatric Evaluation of Adults Guideline (2006), 46, available online at http://www.psychiatryonline.com/pracGuide/loadGuidelinePdf.aspx?file=PsychEval2ePG_04-28-06.

Chapter 9: The Missing Skill

1. Ramin Mojtabai and Mark Olfson, "National Trends in Psychotherapy by Office-Based Psychiatrists," *Archives of General Psychiatry* 65 (2008):962–970.

2. "Study: Many Psychiatrists Do Little More Than Write Prescriptions" August 4, 2008, Fox News.com, http://www.foxnews.com/story/0,2933,397441,00.html.

3. Charles Barber, *Comfortably Numb: How Psychiatry Is Medicating a Nation* (New York: Pantheon, 2008).

4. For a brief classic book on psychoanalysis, see Paul Brenner, *An Elementary Textbook of Psychoanalysis*, rev. ed. (New York: Anchor Books, 1974).

5. Ilana Rabinowitz, ed., *Inside Therapy* (New York: St. Martin's Griffin, 1998), xxiv.

6. For a comprehensive textbook, see Glen Gabbard, *Psychodynamic Psychiatry in Clinical Practice* (4th ed.) (Washington D.C.: American Psychiatric Publishing, Inc., 2005). For a shorter book, see Michael Franz Basch, *Doing Psychotherapy* (New York: Basic Books, 1980).

7. *In Treatment*, HBO.

8. Robert Langreth, "Patient Fix Thyself," *Forbes*, April 9, 2007.

9. For the lay reader, one of the best introductions to the cognitive behavioral therapy approach is David Burns, *Feeling Good: The New Mood Therapy*, reprint ed. (New York: Harper, 1999). For professional readers, an excellent introduction is David Barlow, *Clinical Handbook of Psychological Disorders*, 4th ed. (New York: Guilford Press, 2008).

10. Mantosh Dewan, "Are Psychiatrists Cost-Effective? An analysis of Integrated Versus Split Treatment," *American Journal of Psychiatry* 156 (2) (1999):324–326.

11. According to the survey of a representative sample of American physicians, psychiatrists were by far the least likely to accept managed care contracts. Only 12 percent of other physicians do not accept insurance. Ellyn Boukus, Alwyn Cassil, et al., "A Snapshot of U.S. Physicians: Key Findings from the 2008 Health Tracking Study Physician Survey," Center for Studying Health System Change, Data Bulletin No. 35, September 2009, http://www.hschange.com/CONTENT/1078/.

12. American Society of Clinical Psychopharmacology website, "What Is a Psychopharmacologist?" (http://www.ascpp.org/pages.aspx?PanelID=1&PageName=What_is_Psychopharmacology).

13. Nicholas Kontos, John Querques, et al., "The Problem of the Psychopharmacologist," *Academic Psychiatry* 30 (2006):218–226.

14. Arthur Brody, Sanjaya Saxena et al., "FDG-PET predictors of response to behavioral therapy and pharmacotherapy in obsessive compulsive disorder," *Psychiatry Research* 84(1) (November 9, 1998):1–6.

Chapter 10: Solutions

1. John Bolter, interview with author.

2. Michelle Riba, "APA Armed and Ready to Fight Psychologist-Prescribing Bills," *Psychiatric News* 39 (August 6, 2004).

3. For a review of the literature on physician-extenders, see Richard Cooper and Sandra Stoflet, "Diversity and Consistency: The Challenge of Maintaining Quality in a Multidisciplinary Workforce," *Journal of Health Services Research and Policy* 9, Suppl 1 (2004):39–47.

4. On its Web site, the American College of Neuropsychopharmacology describes itself as the "nation's premier professional society in brain, behavior, and psychopharmacology research." See http://www.acnp.org/aboutus/default.aspx.

5. American College of Neuropsychopharmacology, "DoD Prescribing Psychologists: External Analysis, Monitoring, and Evaluation of the Program and Its

Participants, Final Report," May 1998, http://www.dod.mil/pubs/foi/Prescribe Psychologists.pdf.

6. United States General Accounting Office, "Need for More Prescribing Psychologists Is Not Adequately Justified," April 1997, http://bit.ly/50ZFkK.

7. Peter Cunningham, "Beyond Parity: Primary Care Physicians' Perspectives on Access to Mental Health Care," *Health Affairs* 28 (3) (2009): w490–w501. This article is based on a survey of a nationally representative sample of primary care physicians in 2004–2005. Two thirds of the PCPs reported that they could not get outpatient mental health services for their patients, and this was due primarily to lack of available practitioners, although poor insurance coverage also played a role.

8. Richard Cooper, "Where Is Psychiatry Going and Who Is Going There?" *Academic Psychiatry* 27 (Winter 2003):229–234.

9. Donna Sudak, Judith Beck, et al., "Readiness of Psychiatry Residency Training Programs to Meet the ACGME Requirements in Cognitive-Behavioral Therapy," *Academic Psychiatry* 26 (2002): 96–101.

10. Myrna Weissman, H. Verdeli et al., "National Survey of Psychotherapy Training in Psychiatry, Psychology, and Social Work," *Archives of General Psychiatry* 63 (2006):925–934.

11. American Board of Psychiatry and Neurology, "Psychiatry and Neurology Core Competencies Version 4.1," approved by the ABPN Board of Directors, February 22, 2009, http://www.abpn.com/downloads/core_comp_outlines/core_psych_neuro_v4.1.pdf.

12. American Association of Medical Colleges, National Resident Matching Program, "Charting Outcomes in the Match," 3rd ed., August 2009, http://www.nrmp.org/data/chartingoutcomes2009v3.pdf.

13. Eve Bender, "Public Has Trust Issues with Psychiatrists, Survey Finds," *Psychiatric News* 42 (5) (March 2, 2007):18.

14. Aaron Levin, "Imaging, Genetics on Verge of Transforming Psychiatry," *Psychiatric News* 44 (22) (November 20, 2009):1.

15. Mark Moran, "Psychiatrist Helped Demonstrate Psychotherapy Is Cost-Effective," *Psychiatric News* 44 (22) (November 20, 2009): 1.

ACKNOWLEDGMENTS

Since this book is part memoir, the list of people who have helped me write it is vast. First there is my family. My wife, Tammy Bottner, my son, Ari, and my daughter, Sophia, have allowed *Unhinged* to become a fifth family member for the past two years, and I am grateful for their support and their tolerance. My father, Paul Carlat, a psychiatrist, has been a mentor and unflagging supporter through various endeavors, and is one of the few truly integrative practitioners in the field. My brother-in-law, Richard Naimark, has contributed to this book by representing the model of the wise, down-to-earth psychiatrist for his many grateful patients.

I am indebted to the following colleagues who took time to discuss various topics that found their way into the book. Some of them would agree with the arguments of *Unhinged*, while others would strenuously disagree, but either way our conversations helped me appreciate the nuances of some thorny topics. For this I thank Shahram Ahari, Marc Agronin, Claudia Baldassano, Stan Berman, Katherine Blake, John Bolter, Doug Bremner, Howard Brody, Bernard Carroll, Richard Cooper, Lisa Cosgrove, Larry Diller, David Fassler, Michael First, Allen Frances, Michael Freeman, Ruth Fritz, Adriane Fugh-Berman, Glen Gabbard, Lawrence Gelb, Nassir Ghaemi, Brian Greenfield, Mark Hauser, Victoria Hendrick, Dilip Jeste, Jerome Kassirer, David Kupfer, Alan Lyman, Theo Manschrek, John Miller, Steve Nissen, David Osser, Ron Pies, Darrel Regier, Robert Rubin, Joel Rubinstein, Jim Sabin, Sally Satel, Jim Slayton, Robert Spitzer, Tom Stossel, Nada Stotland, Paul Summergrad, Erick Turner, Robert Wallerstein, Scott Waterman, and Mark Zimmerman.

The members of the editorial board of my monthly newsletter, *The Carlat Psychiatry Report*, have always kept me honest in my more academic writing: Ronald Albucher, Richard Gardiner, Ivan Goldberg, Alan Lyman, Robert Mick, Michael Posternak, Glen Spielmans, and Marcia Zuckerman.

A number of talented health-care journalists, bloggers, and policy makers have contributed to this book, either through thought-provoking conversation or via their reporting. These include David Armstrong, Shannon Brownlee, Ben Carey, Mary Carmichael, Alan Coukell, Philip Dawdy, Marcia Hams, Gardiner Harris, Jeanne Lenzer, Kevin O'Reilly, Kate Peterson, Roy Poses, Gary Schwitzer, Ed Silverman, Paul Thacker, Duff Wilson, and Jun Yan. I thank Ilena Silverman of *The New York Times Magazine* and Mark Horowitz of *Wired* magazine for their masterful editing of articles that provided some material for the chapters on hired guns and the seductions of technology.

My agent, Rafe Sagalyn, served in the dual roles of idea man and personal coach as I searched for a writing project that I could sink my teeth into, and my editor at the Free Press, Emily Loose, amazed me with her comprehensive understanding of every single issue I covered in the book. My assistant, Linsey Mason, provided the organizing principle in my professional life without which this book would still be no more than an outline.

Finally, several friends helpfully read early drafts of chapters or listened to my ideas: Brian Egolf, Rowen Hochstedler, Susan Hochstedler, Leslie Joseph, Jesse Kalfel, Bob Videyko, and Ian Wallis.

INDEX

ABOUT THE AUTHOR

Dr. Daniel Carlat is on the faculty of Tufts Medical School, and did his psychiatric training at Harvard Medical School and Massachusetts General Hospital, where he was chief resident of the inpatient psychiatric unit. He has published several professional books and articles, and is currently the editor in chief of the *Carlat Psychiatry Report* (http://www.thecarlatreport.com), a monthly newsletter read by clinicians throughout the United States. He is also an occasional contributor to the *New York Times*, where he has published articles on psychiatric and medical topics. He can be reached at drcarlat@comcast.net.